Superfoods

The Food and Medicine
of the Future

DAVID WOLFE

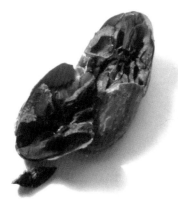

North Atlantic Books
Berkeley, California

Published by
North Atlantic Books   Cover design by Suzanne Albertson
P.O. Box 12327   Book design by Brad Greene
Berkeley, California 94712

Cover photo of David Wolfe by Lesley Bohm.
    All other photo credits can be found on page 313.

Printed in the United States of America

Superfoods: The Food and Medicine of the Future is sponsored by the Society for the Study of Native Arts and Sciences, a nonprofit educational corporation whose goals are to develop an educational and cross-cultural perspective linking various scientific, social, and artistic fields; to nurture a holistic view of arts, sciences, humanities, and healing; and to publish and distribute literature on the relationship of mind, body, and nature.

North Atlantic Books' publications are available through most bookstores. For further information, visit our website at www.northatlanticbooks.com or call 800-733-3000.

Library of Congress Cataloging-in-Publication Data

Wolfe, David.
    Superfoods : the food and medicine of the future / David Wolfe.
        p. cm.
    ISBN 978-1-55643-776-2 (trade pbk.)
    1. Functional foods. 2. Raw food diet. I. Title.
    QP144.F85W65 2009
    613.2'6—dc22
                                                            2009000596

4 5 6 7 8 9 10 11 UNITED 15 14 13 12 11

This book is dedicated
to my Mom—the best mom ever!

☺

Acknowledgments

I would like to thank the following individuals for their direct or indirect contribution to the extraordinary project that became this book:

Mike Adams

Steve Adler

Sandy "Chocolate Face" Brzozowski

Dereme Church

Dandelion

Groovinda Dasi

Len Foley

Juliana Garske

Lucien Gauthier

Michele Gauthier

Rebecca Gauthier

Nick Good

Angela Hartman

Camille "Super Goji Girl" Perrin

Erin Sojourner

Mitch Wallis

Robert "Ra" Weismandel

Richard Grossinger, Doug Reil, Philip Smith, Anne Connolly, and the entire team at North Atlantic Books

Table of Contents

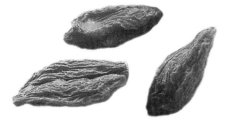

Introduction

Why Superfoods? What Are Superfoods?

A new day is dawning on the world of nutrition. Our nutrition potential has finally caught up to our technology. Shipping, communication, computers, and increased knowledge about nutrition are allowing us to access incredible quality food products from around the planet in a way that had heretofore been impossible or simply unknown.

More and more people are opening up to organic foods and natural health. The organic food movement is taking grocery store chains by storm. We are approaching a critical mass of consumers shifting their purchasing power toward organic products. Would you like to join this leading edge of discovery and find out how to eat the healthiest foods possible?

These special foods fall into three ancient food groups that we are rediscovering in our present-day culture:

1. *Living, raw plant foods:* These are important everyday foods that include most fruits, vegetables, nuts, seeds, seaweeds, sprouts, grasses, fresh herbs, and fermented foods (e.g., sauerkraut). Living, raw plant foods and raw diets are the subject of my previous books *The Sunfood Diet Success System* and *Eating for Beauty.*

2. *Superfoods:* These include foods that have a dozen or more unique properties, not just one or two. For example, the goji berry is a source of complete protein, immune-stimulating polysaccharides, liver-cleansing betaine, anti-aging sesquiterpenes, antioxidants, over twenty trace minerals, and much, much more.

3. *Superherbs:* These include herbs that have super tonic and adaptogenic properties as well as many other unique gifts. For example,

the reishi mushroom helps support a healthy immune system, heart, lungs, and kidneys, and assists with rejuvenating brain and connective tissue. Another example, cat's claw *(uña de gato)*, a superherb from Peru, contains a monoamine oxidase inhibitor that makes you feel happier and has properties that help your immune system fight off viruses. Superherbs will be the subject of a future book, and are contained in some of my recipes here.

We truly live in a time of unprecedented abundance. Having access to and knowledge of the world's greatest superfoods, superherbs, and living, raw plant foods at this level of quality is a first in human history. In spite of the seemingly insurmountable problems of civilization, we are still making progress in becoming healthier and more self-aware beings. We are finally discovering the power of adding into our diet an entirely new class of foods that benefits everyone with maximum nutrition, protein, flavor, health, energy, as well as minimum calories and no trans-fatty acids.

It is becoming clearer that to achieve the best health ever, the best relationship with food ever, and to have the most fun with our food ever, we must consume superfoods, superherbs, and raw and living food cuisine. In doing so, we will find that our desire for less healthy foods will fall away naturally because we no longer find them as enjoyable.

Of these three food classes, superfoods are the most important and the focus of each page before you. Superfoods comprise a specific set of edible, incredibly nutritious plants that are not entirely classifiable as foods nor are they entirely classifiable medicines (such as herbs).

Superfoods are both a food and a medicine; they have elements of both. They are a class of the most potent, super-concentrated, and nutrient-rich foods on the planet—they have more bang for the buck than our usual foods. Extremely tasty and satisfying, superfoods have the ability to tremendously increase the vital force and energy of one's body, and are the

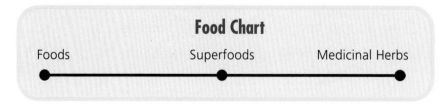

Food Chart

| Foods | Superfoods | Medicinal Herbs |

optimum choice for improving overall health, boosting the immune system, elevating serotonin production, enhancing sexuality, and cleansing and alkalizing the body. Superfoods meet and exceed all our protein requirements, our vitamin and mineral requirements, glyconutrient (essential polysaccharide sugar) requirements, essential fatty acid requirements, immune system requirements, and so much more. Nourishing us at the deepest level possible, they are the true fuel of today's "superhero." Superfoods make having The Best Day Ever fast, easy, fresh, and fun!

Superfoods are a major focal point of nutrition because they not only help nourish the brain, bones, muscles, skin, hair, nails, heart, lungs, liver, kidneys, reproductive system, pancreas, and immune system, they also, over the long term, correct imbalances and help to guide us toward a more natural and aboriginal diet. Consuming superfoods makes it dramatically easier to achieve your ideal weight, diet, and food habits. Superfoods will ease you into detoxification and the transition to more healthy foods—all without willpower! Additionally, superfoods help you do this without having to take dead vitamin and mineral supplements.

The scientific studies included in this book highlight some of the ongoing discoveries about superfoods as an essential part of a balanced diet. Superfoods allow us to get more nutrition with less eating. Most of us have had many experiences of eating all day just to keep our blood sugar up, yet we received very little nourishment in the process. We know that most of the conventional foods and fast foods today are nothing but empty calories.

Organic fruits, vegetables, nuts, seeds, sprouts, and other healthy plant foods are a very important part of our diet, but they do not compare to the nutrient density of superfoods. In my own diet, I eat fruits and vegetables primarily for flavor, fiber, and bulk, not for deep levels of nutrition. When it comes to real nutrition, only superfoods can meet and exceed all requirements.

Eating superfoods is a way to guarantee that you will get the nutrients you require to be healthy all the years of your life. Because superfoods are natural, they provide an abundance of synergistic elements in their natural state that work together in the human body in ways that scientists have not yet begun to fully comprehend. Scientists have yet to isolate and name all the nutrients found in plants. What we understand about nutrition by listing vitamins, minerals, protein, fats, and carbohydrates on the sides of packages does not give us a complete picture. The common vitamins and minerals that we know of are not the only nutrients that matter. At this point we know of over a thousand vitamins, minerals, amino acids, short-chain sugars, polysaccharides, fats, oils, enzymes, coenzymes, antioxidants, and other substances that contribute to optimum health. In the years ahead, we will discover even more.

Due to the depletion of nutrients in conventional (and to some degree, even organic) foods, we have continued to turn toward new possibilities for whole and balanced nutrition. Superfoods represent an awesome piece of the nutrition puzzle, as they are great sources of clean, hormone-free, pesticide, and chemical-free:

Protein	Vitamins
Minerals	Enzymes
Antioxidants	Coenzymes
Good fats and oils	Essential fatty acids
Essential amino acids	Polysaccharides
Glyconutrients	

Superfoods can and should be consumed in raw and organic form, because decades of research have demonstrated that living, organic raw food is superior in vitamin content, enzymes, coenzymes, protein, minerals, glyconutrients, and many other elements of nutrition. Even chimpanzees in zoos will select fresh, organic raw food in preference to other foods. Nature provides us with raw food. It is time to take advantage of all the scientific breakthroughs in the field of living enzymes! The superfoods mentioned in this book are loaded to the hilt with enzymes. They are, for the most part, the most enzyme-rich foods found in nature. They restore enzyme deficiencies and create enzyme abundance. This is the primary reason why superfoods should be eaten raw and why nearly all the recipes found in this book are made with raw foods, superfoods, and superherbs.

Because superfoods have a high level of inner vitality and life-force energy, they can be grown organically without chemicals or artificial fertilizers. Superfoods are not only great for you, they also help the

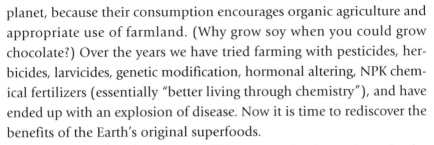

planet, because their consumption encourages organic agriculture and appropriate use of farmland. (Why grow soy when you could grow chocolate?) Over the years we have tried farming with pesticides, herbicides, larvicides, genetic modification, hormonal altering, NPK chemical fertilizers (essentially "better living through chemistry"), and have ended up with an explosion of disease. Now it is time to rediscover the benefits of the Earth's original superfoods.

Our focus within these pages will be upon what I perceive to be the top ten superfoods, as well as an additional group of "honorable mentions." The top ten superfoods are:

Goji berries
Cacao
Maca
Bee products (honey, bee pollen, propolis, and royal jelly)
Spirulina
AFA blue-green algae
Marine phytoplankton
Aloe vera
Hempseed
Coconuts and coconut products

Adding Superfoods to Your Diet

Too many of us live in a state of poor health, lethargy, and moderate obesity. Life continues on, yet slowly we lose our full capabilities, and our quality of life decreases in spite of material successes. Underlying issues of back pain, headaches, joint inflammation, arthritis, threats of cancer, skin problems, and insomnia begin to become more prominent. One day continuous chronic pain sets in as the discomfort increases. Doctor visits and surgeries only serve to mask symptoms or remove diseased tissue and fail to root out the underlying cause of the symptoms and poor health. Eventually the will to live becomes exhausted.

I am absolutely certain that nobody wants this to happen to them. I am also absolutely certain that this fate will befall nearly everyone unless each individual does something specifically about it. I am 100 percent sure it is possible at any age to change our destiny into one of pain-free, vibrant health by intelligently utilizing the power of superfoods, super-herbs, raw and living foods, and holistic healing technologies. We can alter our course and remake ourselves right now at this very second by eating the best foods ever—superfoods. Superfoods are true health foods. They are known to improve the severity and symptoms of nearly every major disease condition known, including:

Allergies	Hepatitis
Arthritis	Herpes (I, II, Epstein-Barr)
Asthma	High blood pressure
Atherosclerosis	HIV infections
Attention Deficit Disorder (ADD)	Hypoglycemia
Cancer (all types)	Insomnia
Chronic fatigue	Multiple sclerosis
Depression	Nervous system disorders
Diabetes (types 1 and 2)	Poor immunity
Eczema	Psoriasis
Fibromyalgia	Skin disorders
Heart disease	

Manufacturing a New Immune System

As you read this book, you will begin to see a common pattern among superfoods: They all actively work to "pre-load" the immune system with the raw materials necessary to maintain a healthy immune system and to mount healthy immune responses.

If you are paying close attention to health information worldwide, you have probably picked up on an important trend: increasingly, it is all about the immune system. With a well-chosen, organic, raw, plant-based diet, fresh raw materials provided by superfoods, and the immediate manufacture of specific immune-system weapons assisted by superherbs—these include the world's greatest herbs, such as *pau d'arco* and cat's claw from the Amazon, the medicinal mushrooms (chaga, reishi, maitake, shiitake, lion's mane, coriolus, cordyceps, etc.), astragalus, schizandra berries, nettles, horsetail, and dozens of other superherbs—

we stand a chance to improve our health in a way that has never been available to us in the past.

Detoxification: Breaking Syndrome X

Nearly everyone raised on a modern American or European diet has consumed mineral-deficient food, foods sprayed with pesticides, antibiotic-treated meat, hormonally altered dairy products, refined sugar, refined grains, and refined salt. In some cases, the toxic load can be overwhelming, causing a metabolic syndrome designated "Syndrome X." Syndrome X is the inability to lose weight, accompanied by a dysfunctional immune system and low energy. Adding organic raw and living foods, superfoods, and superherbs to one's diet can break the hold of Syndrome X, allow one to lose weight and achieve an ideal state of health.

When we begin adding organic, raw, natural superfoods, superherbs, and foods, an astounding metamorphosis can occur and Syndrome X can finally be turned around. Yet we must be very careful not to go faster than our bodies can handle. To be able to handle the metabolic change that occurs through inner cleaning, you need to transition at your own pace and begin where you are. Gradually move up that pace when you can.

The Ideal and the Noble

The ultimate conclusion of "you are what you eat" is that everything you put into your mouth is going to affect your mind, body, and spirit.

Humans have had to adapt to many types of foods over the course of time. In situations where food resources were scarce, those humans who could make-do on what was available were more likely to survive. There has been genetic pressure toward adaptability of diet. Surviving long enough after eating something to let others know that you are still alive, however, is no criterion with which to ascertain what is an ideal diet.

With superfoods, for the first time ever, we get to experiment for ourselves with dietary ideals. We get to eat noble foods and activate our imaginations with the ideals that those superfoods generate within us.

The whole concept of self-healing really revolves around removing poisons, toxins, chemicals, and pesticides from our bodies while ridding ourselves of excess fat. Superfoods in particular contain substantially more nutrients (minerals, enzymes, polysaccharides, protein, and healthy fats and oils) than cooked and processed chemically grown foods. The higher energy content of superfoods delivers more goodies to our cells, which are then capable of throwing off toxins they previously lacked the energy to eliminate. This process is detoxification.

Acidity and Weight Loss

More and more scientific articles and books are being written about the "acid-alkaline" balance and its effect on nutrition. Generally, with a poor diet, the inner environment of our bodies becomes more acidic, creating a breeding ground of disease-causing microbes and organisms. Three main food classes are needed to counteract this progression into acidity and chronic illness: green superfoods, green vegetables, and herbs.

High acidity is usually the primary contributing cause of being overweight. If the body state is acidic, then the body will hold extra water to dilute the acids. Also, the body will store excess acids in the fat tissue, which leads to cellulite and weight gain.

It is important to understand that, when you detoxify, you may release acids from your fat cells and tissues. If these acids are not met with highly alkaline minerals bombarding the body from every direction in the form of green superfoods, green vegetables, and herbs, then problems can arise, ranging from fatigue, hot flashes, mood swings, and bone mineral loss to dental problems such as cavities. Eating superfoods, vegetables, and herbs is essential! It is our insurance policy for health and long life.

At this point, pretty much everyone knows that diets and typical diet strategies don't work. Well then ... what does work?

It is human nature that we do not like being denied things. As soon as you tell a child "No," they are immediately finding a way to "Yes." They will do what they want if they can get away with it. This habit never changes. We do the same thing as adults. Battling this quirk of human nature is like trying to stop the sun from setting or rising, or the planets from moving.

Instead, we have to get in alignment with our true nature. What does that mean? How about this: Instead of taking foods away from people, how about adding foods in? How about turning people on to all kinds of new food flavors, tastes, textures, colors, and combinations? Is it possible that the "good" food will be so good, and will make us feel so good, that we'll naturally move away from the "bad" food? In my experience, the answer is YES. In this way, the transformation in diet is accomplished without trying. Everything happens gracefully. That is the idea behind this book; that is the essence of superfood nutrition. We put the focus on all the great-tasting, super-healthy foods there are for us to discover and enjoy. To me, the superfood diet is the best diet ever because it requires only adding new gorgeous foods into my lifestyle at a pace that I enjoy and that feels great.

Any of the superfoods can be added into anyone's diet. Simply find the ones you like and start guzzling them. Get out a blender and make entirely new types of shakes and smoothies out of superfoods. Make superfood treats and desserts. Create superfood salad dressings. Design superfood trail mixes. Make a tea out of your favorite superherbs and blend the tea with superfoods.

The superfood diet approximates what I perceive as the underlying approach of the great Taoist herbal masters of Chinese history, which is to add in the most powerful superfoods and superherbs, knowing that you

Superfood Seeds

The goal of this book is to support you in selecting the healthiest super-foods on the planet while providing new options of what you can grow in your garden. As long as we are going to grow something, why not grow superfoods along with our tomatoes and lettuce?

The logical next question is: Where do I get seeds for superfoods, or baby superfood plants? The answer is that they are usually contained in the food itself. For example, we recently did a planting experiment on a sample of organic goji berries. We planted sixty-four goji berries (tearing them open to allow the seeds to be exposed to the soil). Of these, every one sprouted. That's a 100 percent sprouting ratio!

will naturally lose interest in the unhealthier foods in your diet. Superfoods also go a long way toward making us more balanced in behavior and demeanor due to remineralization of our tissues and the superior, well-rounded nutrition that superfoods provide.

When you bring superfoods into your body, your energy changes, and as a result your focus of attention will shift as well. It is likely that you will reassess your values (what you consider important). You may see the world with more energy behind your eyes: with that added boost, it becomes easier to live in a state of appreciation. Over time, you will likely perceive the world as a more amazing place than ever before, because you will feel better more often. I eat superfoods every day, and they make me feel the best ever, always!

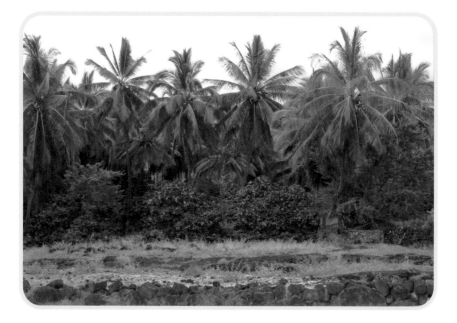

A Note on the Recipes

The recipes in this book range from beginner and intermediate to advanced, for all levels of superfood enthusiasts. Because some of the ingredients may be new to you, I have included a glossary of these ingredients at the back of the book to help acquaint you with any unfamiliar terms.

Some of the items in these recipes are exotic and unique. Online shopping makes them easily accessible. Depending on your budget, you may choose smaller or larger sizes of the listed superfoods, superherbs, and supplements in order to give them a try. Prices on these items vary, so spend your money wisely, experiment, and play. Remember, a little bit of these ingredients goes a long way.

The kitchen appliances referenced in the recipes are recommended but not required. For example, a high-speed blender is mentioned in numerous recipes. This type of blender commands a significantly higher price in the marketplace than a typical home blender. I have been using the Vita-Mix® blender since 1980 and I know they are durable and worth the investment. A simple home blender may be substituted for a high-speed blender in the recipes, even though they are not quite as great. When it makes sense for you, purchasing a high-speed blender will make superfood recipes even easier to create.

Another appliance worth discussing is the dehydrator. I recommend Excalibur dehydrators because I have been using them regularly since 1998. I have never found any other dehydrator that I enjoyed using as much or that worked as effectively. If the Excalibur is outside of your range right now, then using a stove at low temperatures is recommended for dehydration purposes.

Enjoy all the superfood recipes and join us in enjoying the prosperous abundance found in superfoods—the food of the future!

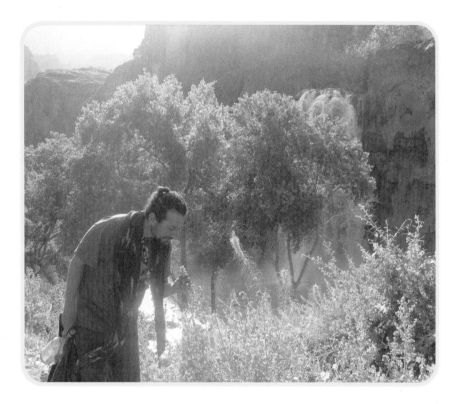

The Top
10 Superfoods

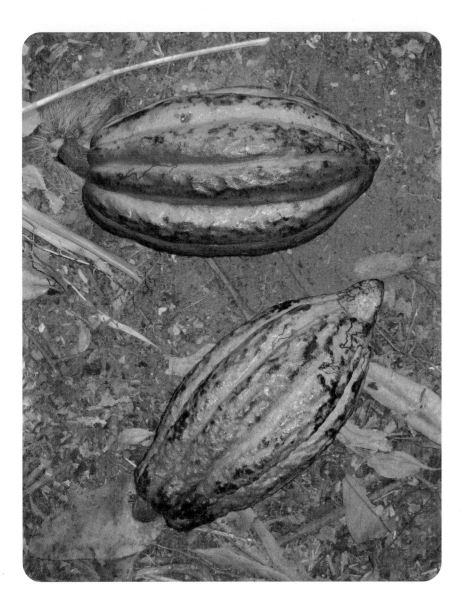

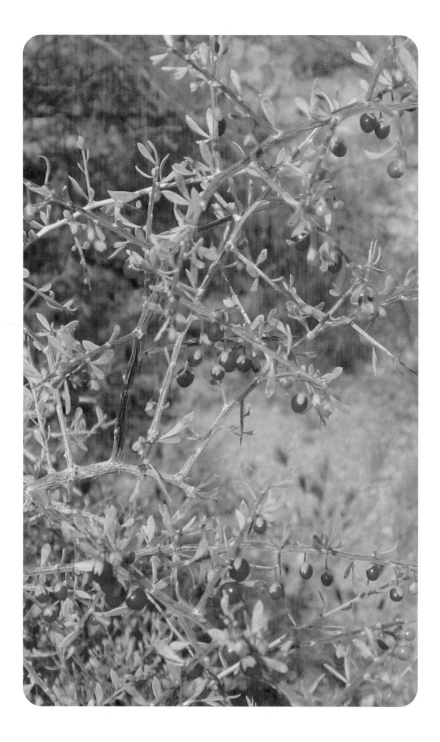

Goji Berries
Fountain of Youth

Latin Names:

Major Asian varieties: *Lycium barbarum, Lycium chinensis*

Major American varieties: *Lycium andersonii, Lycium berlandieri, Lycium brevipes, Lycium californicum, Lycium carolinianum, Lycium cooperi, Lycium exsertum, Lycium fremontii, Lycium halimifolium, Lycium macrodon, Lycium pallidum, Lycium parishii, Lycium puberlum, Lycium torreyi* (*Lycium* is also spelled *Lyceum,* depending on the reference text or web site)

Common Names:

Goji Berry, Wolfberry, Boxthorn, Matrimony Vine, Desert Thorn

Superfood Type:

Berry (fruit)

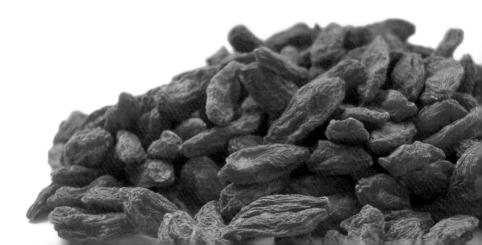

The following parts of the goji berry bush have also been used in herbal preparations or as food:

Seeds
Flowers
Leaves
Roots

History, Facts, and Legends

Goji berries grow on a bush that develops like a vine when grown in the shade. At the very largest, the goji bush will grow six feet tall and will have a radius of around three feet. The ovate leaves range in length from half an inch to four inches depending on location and variety. Red striations are sometimes seen in the bark of the plant. Although not specifically a thorny plant like a rose, some American goji berry varieties can develop some thornlike stems. During the nonflowering seasons (summer, fall, and winter), the goji berry bush may lose some or all of its leaves, which makes it more difficult to recognize. In spring, however, the leaves fill out beautifully and pale-white to purple flowers enrich the plant, usually beginning in March in the northern hemisphere. Following the flower pollination, fruit berries will soon follow. Goji berries range in color from pale yellow to dark sunfire orange to deep red. Sometimes the raisin-sized goji berries are oblong, like footballs. I have even seen goji berries that are shaped like small peppers. Often the berries are entirely spherical.

There are an estimated eighty-five species of goji berry in Asia and fifteen species in North and Central America. It is possible, based on this geographic dispersion, that the goji berry was brought to North America by groups who migrated from Asia, either by boat or across the Bering Land Bridge.

The goji berries of Asia and America are remarkably similar. The history of the Asian varieties is better documented, researched, and consecrated in legend and lore, but both the Asian and American goji berry varieties deserve special attention because their histories and health-giving properties are so rich.

All goji berries that I have studied and grown are remarkably adaptable. The goji berries grow as wonderfully in harsh, dry deserts as they do in the tropics. Goji berries also tolerate freezing winters and have been recorded to grow well in such places as Nova Scotia and British Columbia. Perhaps most interesting is that goji berries can handle daily swings in temperature as great as 40 degrees Fahrenheit.

The goji berry was categorized under the Linnaean Latin categorization system under the genus *Lycium* (or *Lyceum*). From its Greek root, the word *Lyceum* means "school of learning." And that is what the masters of Chinese herbalism believed the goji berry could provide. Legend has it that one can tune into a pharmacopeia of herbal data contained within the plant simply by eating goji berries. Further, some believe that if one studies, grows, and eats the goji berry, it is able to teach you the fundamental principles of Chinese herbalism.

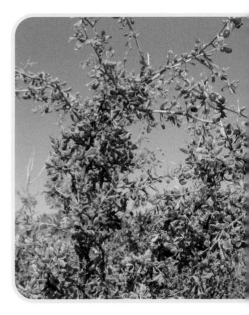

Asian Goji Berries

Because of the goji berry's extraordinary nutrient value, rich red-orange color, and pleasant, full-bodied taste, the Chinese, Mongolian, and Tibetan peoples have been growing the alkaline goji berry plant for an estimated five thousand years. To preserve the fruit, it is often dried until similar to a dry raisin in texture.

In Chinese tradition, the spirit or *deva* of the goji bush is often represented as a young, virile female who is—interestingly—not of Asian ethnicity. Ningxia Province in China, where goji berries are primarily grown, has more centenarians than the rest of the country, and the residents of the province age more gracefully. They are more active, healthy, and vibrant than elderly people in Western countries. Of course, goji berries are a key ingredient in their healthy diet. The Chinese hold a strong belief that this fruit can significantly extend life.

The famed Li Qing Yuen, whom legend has it popularized both goji berries and ginseng, and is said to have lived to the age of 252 years (1678–1930), consumed goji berries daily. The life of Li Qing Yuen is the most documented case of extreme longevity known. The legend of Li

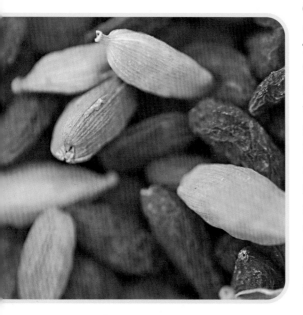

Qing Yuen says that when Li was eleven years old he met three Taoist sages who were purported to be over three hundred years old. They taught Li about spring water and the science and fine art of longevity, proper diet, and herbalism. Later in his life, at the age of fifty, he was said to have met another Taoist sage who told Li he was five hundred years old. When Li inquired about the secret of his extreme longevity, the sage taught him to consume a goji berry soup each day.

Li Qing Yuen is said to have given a lecture at the University of Beijing at the age of two hundred. When the emperor of China discovered such a long-lived person within the empire, he invited Li to the royal court. Within a few months of living in Beijing, Li Qing Yuen was dead, apparently either from eating the processed food provided by the royal kitchen or from exposure to the toxicity of the city.

Even if Li Qing Yuen's longevity is just a myth, it does demonstrate a recognized relationship in the culture between the goji berry and longevity.

By the way, as far as I have been able to uncover from studying the life of Li Qing Yuen for over a decade, his daily tea consisted of goji berries, ginseng, and reishi mushrooms. You can make this tea at home and it is delightful. I often use wild reishi mushrooms that I pick from the forest behind my home.

The famed elixir of longevity in Chinese medicine is supposed to have consisted of goji berries and flowers picked in spring, leaves picked in the spring or summer, and the root picked in autumn. All of these mixed together into a super tonic were said to keep one young indefinitely.

Goji berries are also grown in Tibet and have been recognized by the Tibetan School of Medicine in Lhasa as a superfood for twenty-five hundred years. The *Lycium barbarum* variety of the goji berry is said to have originally been from Tibet. Only the goji berries packed under the *Tibet Authentic* brand are actually grown in Tibet. Other advertised "Tibetan" goji berries are grown in Mongolia or China.

American Goji Berries

American goji berry varieties are concentrated mostly in the desert Southwest of the United States (Arizona, California, Colorado, Utah, New Mexico, Texas) with some species also present in the western deserts of Mexico and South America. The goji berry was an important food source for nearly all Native American tribes in the desert Southwest including the Hopi, Apache, Supai, Hohokam, Pima, Anasazi, Navajo, Zuni, and many others.

The great Apache, Geronimo, was born in one of the most dense, wild goji-berry regions of America. The Apaches subsisted on goji berries, corn, saguaro cactus fruit, barrel cactus fruit, red-seeded watermelons, wild walnuts, wild apples, wild grapes, wild game and fish, green herbs, some domesticated beans, herbs such as devil's claw, and spring water. The tribe was known to possess astounding strength, agility, longevity, and survival skills.

Benefits

Overview

The goji berry is an "adaptogen," a term used in the world of medicinal plants to describe a substance with a combination of therapeutic actions on the human body. An adaptogen invigorates and strengthens the system while helping the body to deal more easily with stress by supporting the adrenal glands. In the Chinese medicinal system, the goji berry is known to harmonize and increase the *jing* energy of the adrenals and kidneys, resulting in enhanced stamina, strength, longevity, and sexual energy.

Overall, goji berries boost immune function, increase alkalinity and vitality, provide liver protection, improve eyesight and blood quality, deliver anti-aging compounds, and possess a number of additional outstanding qualities.

Although often recommended for such chronic conditions as liver or kidney disorders, weak joints and legs, lower back problems, dizziness and tinnitus, headaches, insomnia, hypertension, tuberculosis, and impotence, goji berries are not used for treating illness or poor health as such. Their main health benefit is to nourish the body—to support the body in healing itself by providing a startling array of extraordinary nutrients.

Goji berries are perhaps the most nutritionally rich berry-fruit on the planet. They taste delicious and are well-balanced for nearly all body types, blood types, and metabolisms. They are a complete protein source, and contain nineteen different amino acids (on par with bee pollen) and all eight essential amino acids (such as adrenal-supporting phenylalanine and serotonin-building tryptophan). Goji berries can contain twenty-one or more trace minerals (the main ones being zinc, iron, copper, calcium, germanium, selenium, and phosphorus) as well as vitamins B1, B2, B6, and vitamin E.

Contrary to Internet marketing claims, the dried goji berry is not a rich source of vitamin C. I have had different batches of dried organic goji berries tested three times for vitamin C by reputable labs and found that the content was nearly zero. At this time I have been unable to find any laboratory reports indicating that either dried or fresh goji berries contain a significant quantity of vitamin C.

Depending on variety and growing conditions, mature goji berries can contain about 11 mg of blood-building iron per 100 grams (2–3 handfuls) as well as beta-sitosterol (an anti-inflammatory agent), linoleic acid (an essential fatty acid), anti-aging sesquiterpenoids (cyperone, solavetivone), liver-healing betaine (0.1 percent), and antioxidant tetraterpenoids (zeaxanthin, physalin). Goji berries are some of the highest antioxidant-containing foods in the world. They typically contain two to four times the amount of antioxidants found in blueberries.

Goji berries contain long-chain sugars known as polysaccharides that fortify the immune system. The short- and long-chain sugars that the goji berry contains include: D-rhamnose, D-xylose, D-arabinose, D-fucose,

D-glucose, and D-galactose. About 36 percent of the sugars found in domesticated goji berries are the interesting long-chain sugar polysaccharides. The percentage is greater in wild goji-berry varieties.

As we age, we produce less and less Human Growth Hormone (HGH). Decreasing levels of HGH have been linked to symptoms of aging. Goji berries are the only food known to help stimulate the human body to produce more HGH naturally. This factor alone makes the goji berry perhaps the world's greatest anti-aging superfood.

Longevity and Healthy Hormones

The great macrobiotic nutritionist Michio Kushi used to say, "Eat according to your purpose." If at least part of your purpose is longevity and vitality, then the goji berry is the superfood for you. Evidence from every direction indicates that the goji berry is the leading longevity superfood in the world. It has been nicknamed "the longevity fruit." Researchers who study medicinal plants have identified a variety of nutrients in the goji berry that may help people enjoy longer and healthier lives.

A seventy-year-old produces only one-tenth of the amount of Human Growth Hormone (HGH) generated by a twenty-year-old. This decline parallels physical deterioration, such as lower levels of energy, muscle wasting, and a tendency to store more body fat. Boosting the natural production of growth hormone helps us feel, look, and function like a more youthful person. Goji berries help our bodies do this in several interesting ways.

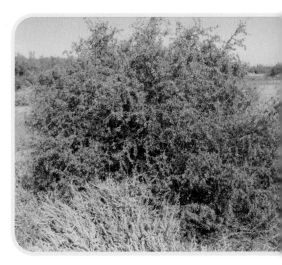

There is evidence that goji berries increase longevity because they are high in sesquiterpenoids. Sesquiterpenoids have anti-inflammatory properties. They stimulate the pituitary and pineal glands thus increasing the glandular production of HGH. Human Growth Hormone is a master hormone that influences the level of all hormones in the body. Remember, as we age, HGH decreases. In order to achieve great longevity, we have to maintain HGH production. The goji berry is the only food known that is a confirmed secretagogue (a secretagogue is a compound that stimulates HGH).

The presence of certain amino acids in the goji berry may also promote the production of HGH. The goji berry is a rich source of l-glutamine and l-arginine. These two amino acids work together to boost growth hormone levels in order to revitalize one's appearance and metabolism.

Enhancing Libido and Sexual Function

In Asia, goji berries are traditionally regarded as a strong sexual tonic. In addition, goji berries act as a general tonic to improve overall stamina, mood, and well-being while decreasing the impact of stress on our bod-

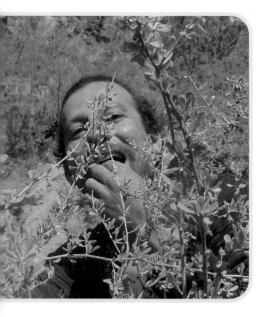

ies. All of these benefits together are conducive to a healthier, richer sex life.

Diminished sexual function is not an inevitable part of aging. A lower sex drive in both men and women can be associated with a decreased production of testosterone. Goji berries help by increasing HGH production, which then facilitates an increase in testosterone production.

Antioxidants

Antioxidants protect our DNA from free radical and radiation damage. DNA damage opens the door to every imaginable illness and accelerates aging. Over the course of time, our DNA is damaged by free radicals, generated as a byproduct of normal metabolism, and by exposure to toxins and radiation.

Although our bodies are equipped to continually repair themselves, they can become overwhelmed by too many free radicals, especially as we age. This results in the premature death of healthy cells, which may contribute to a variety of degenerative diseases and to the accelerated development of mutated cells that can lead to cancer—unless antioxidants counter the onslaught.

The goji berry is nature's richest food source of antioxidant carotenoids (such as beta-carotene—goji berries contain more beta-carotene than carrots). Carotenoids are natural fat-soluble antioxidant pigments.

The carotenoid content of mammal tissue is a statistically significant factor in determining Maximal Life Span Potential (MLSP). For example, a human MLSP of approximately 90 years correlates with a serum carotene level of 50 to 300 micrograms per deciliter while other primates, such as the rhesus monkey, have an MLSP of approximately 34 years correlating with a serum carotene level of 6 to 12 micrograms per deciliter. In essence, it appears that the more carotenoids mammals eat, the longer they will live.

Improving Vision

The goji berry contains two key antioxidants for healthy vision: zeaxanthin and lutein. Free radicals attack the eyes, and zeaxanthin and lutein protect against and help repair such damage.

These antioxidants concentrate themselves at the center of the retina and protect the eye from the most common causes of age-related loss of sight, including macular degeneration, cataracts, and diabetic retinopathy.

Goji berries contain perhaps the highest concentration of the eyesight-improving antioxidant zeaxanthin of any natural superfood or herbal product currently on the market. Zeaxanthin helps heal the membranes of our eyes and also gives them luster and youthfulness. In the Chinese medicinal system, goji berries have been recommended for thousands of years to improve eyesight.

Immune System Booster

There appear to be three major components of the goji berry that improve the immune system: the goji berry polysaccharides (lycium barbarum polysaccharides, or LBPs), beta-carotene, and the mineral germanium.

The goji berry polysaccharides (LBP I, LBP II, LBP III, LBP IV), which are components of the carbohydrate makeup of the goji berry, are world renowned for their ability to improve the immune system and protect cells from genetic mutation.

Beta-carotene appears to enhance thymus gland function and increase interferon's stimulatory action on the immune system. Interferon is a powerful immune-enhancing compound that plays a central role in protection against viral infection.

Research indicates that goji berries contain organic germanium (the goji berry is estimated by Internet sources to contain 124 parts per million of germanium). Germanium has been demonstrated to have cancer-fighting properties. Japanese studies indicate that organic germanium is effective in treating cervical cancer, liver cancer, lung cancer, testicular cancer, and uterine cancer. Like beta-carotene, germanium has been found to induce the production of immune-enhancing interferon.

Hydration

Goji berries—especially wild, fresh goji berries growing in rich, alkaline alluvial soils—contain a tremendous amount of hydrogen. Hydrogen is what is needed to create "hydration." Being hydrated is a function of consuming enough hydrogen; the word "hydro-gen" reveals the science behind its meaning: "hydro" is water, "gen" is generator. In indigenous desert environments where water is scarce, eating goji berries is a critical part of survival.

Supporting Brain and Neurological Health

Goji berries help our bodies produce choline, an essential nutrient that combats free- radical damage linked to neurological degeneration and Alzheimer's disease.

Supporting Cardiovascular Health

Goji berries fight narrowing of the arteries that deliver oxygen and nutrients to all of our cells. Goji berries have the ability to combat a key factor that causes heart disease: oxidized cholesterol. Cholesterol becomes especially dangerous when it oxidizes as a result of free radicals, and the oxidized blood fats attach to artery walls with calcium-forming nanobacteria to form plaques. Our bodies have a built-in defense system against this, an enzyme called superoxide dismutase (SOD). SOD is a super-antioxidant that prevents cholesterol from oxidizing. Chinese research shows that goji berries can increase our production of SOD.

> Goji berries are perhaps the most nutritionally rich berry-fruit on the planet. They taste delicious and are well-balanced for nearly all body types, blood types, and metabolisms.

Keeping Vital Organs Healthy

Goji berries are a tonic adaptogen—they keep our vital organs healthy by balancing blood sugar and enhancing the liver, digestive system, and skin. Goji berry tea has been used in Asia for the treatment of diabetes and to help regulate high blood sugar, which is a precursor to both diabetes and heart disease.

Several types of phytonutrients in the fruit enhance the ability of the liver to detoxify and guard against the organ being damaged by carcinogens and the hepatitis virus. These phytonutrients include betaine, polysaccharides, and antioxidant pigments. Betaine cleans the liver and reduces the toxic amino acid homocysteine (a byproduct of nanobacteria) in the cardiovascular system. Betaine and other goji phytonutrients may be the reason why the goji berry has anti-inflammatory properties.

Goji berry tea is also helpful for all types of digestive problems and can aid in recovery from digestive illnesses such as ulcers and irritable bowel syndrome. Research suggests that the goji berry polysaccharides are responsible for the calming effect on digestion. Goji berries contain fatty acids (including hexadecanoic acid, linoleic acid, beta-elemene, myristic acid, and ethyl hexadecanoate) and Ormus-carrying polysaccharides, which can stimulate collagen production and retain moisture, resulting in younger-looking skin.

What to Look For . . .

Goji Superfood Product Types

The goji berry is a deep red, dried fruit about the same size as a raisin. It tastes somewhat like a cross between a cranberry and a cherry, with an aftertaste that is slightly herbal.

When purchasing dried goji berries, look for the following characteristics:

1. Purchase organic berries. Nonorganic and/or "wild-crafted" berries are mostly sprayed with chemical pesticides and/or sulfur dioxide. Organic goji products are superior in quality, nutrition, and flavor.

2. Select moist berries—but not overly moist, as they may be soaked in sugar water, then re-dried. The goji berry should be reasonably soft and slightly moist. Hard and excessively dry berries should be avoided.

3. With goji berries, size does not count. I have observed no relationship between berry size and quality. Goji berries are often classified into four grades according to size: supreme, first, second, and third grades. The supreme grade has the biggest size, but that does not always equate with the most nutrients.

4. Select berries that have a rich red color, but not unusually so. Unusually red conventionally grown goji berries (that are sold at low prices) may have actually been dyed red with chemicals. Dull goji berries are either old and/or low in antioxidants.

Below is a list of goji products to look for on the Internet or in your health food store or supplement shop:

Dried goji berries
Goji berry extract powder (in bulk bags or capsules)
Goji berry juice (made from goji concentrates)
Goji berry liquid tinctures and extracts (preferably made from fresh, wild goji berries—not dried)
Freshly picked berries

Goji seed oil (topical cosmetic applications)
Raw goji berry chocolate bars, chocolate brittles, and energy bars

How to Use Goji Berries

Because of their history as a tonic adaptogen superfood, goji berries and goji products may be consumed daily. A reasonable daily intake of dried goji berries is 15–45 grams (a handful). There are usually four to six dried berries per gram.

Since the beginning of history, people have used goji berries to make tea, soup, and wine, or simply chewed them like raisins. Goji berries may be used, like other dried fruits, as snacks or mixed in with recipes or smoothies.

There appears to be some truth to the traditional Chinese notion that when dried goji berries are added to other foods or dishes, digestion is improved. Goji berries appear to draw digestive juices into the stomach and intestines. Dr. Iichiroh Ohhira, a Japanese scientist who has invested nearly forty years in studying bacteria, includes friendly bacteria along with the goji berry in his outstanding cultured probiotic formulas.

Organic goji berries can be mixed with cacao nibs and/or many other superfoods, dried fruits, nuts, and seeds to make goji trail mixes. Cacao nibs and goji berries go particularly well. Because of their combined antioxidant content, cacao and goji berries make for excellent air-travel snacks.

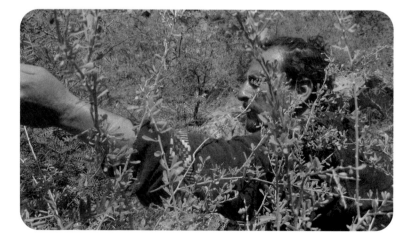

You can blend dried goji berries directly into smoothies, juices, and elixirs. A reasonably strong blender will completely blend the dried goji berries into the beverage.

Goji berries can be soaked and rehydrated in water. Goji water makes for a wonderfully hydrating beverage and can also be used for the base of a soup stock.

Goji berries are an excellent tea additive. Whatever tea you are making, throw ten to twenty goji berries into the mix and notice how they take the bitter edge off of medicinal herbs and how they accentuate and synergize all the tea ingredients. Also try drinking goji berry tea all by itself. An iced goji berry tea is delightful in the summer. Drinking the tea is an easy way to make goji berry polysaccharides more available to the human body, as they extract from the berries into hot water.

Dried goji berries should be stored in a dry sealable bag or container. They will absorb a lot of moisture if they are open to the air.

Goji Berry Recipes

Goji Water

I like to soak my gojis in water to rehydrate them, but only use the soak water for my smoothie base. As a recipe:

1 large handful of goji berries

3 cups water

Soak at least 2–4 hours in room-temperature water and occasionally stir. Pour through strainer to remove berries. Use goji water as base for smoothie.

Add to the goji water:

1–2 cups of your favorite berries

1 tbsp. raw honey or yacon syrup

1/2 vanilla bean, scrape out the seeds

Blend all ingredients in a high-powered blender until smooth. You can also add favorite superfoods like hempseed, chocolate powder, protein powder, or green superfood powder.

Electrolyte Lemon Goji Lemon Aid

- 1 cup goji berries soaked in 1/2 gallon of water 2 to 4 hours. Strain through mesh and use soak water
- 1 lemon, freshly juiced
- 1 pinch Himalayan salt

Lightly sweeten if desired.

Goji Balls

- 2 cups dried goji berries blended in a high-speed blender*
- 1 cup tocotrienols
- 2 tbsp. coconut oil
- 2 tbsp. raw honey
- 1 handful cacao nibs
- 1 heaping tbsp. chocolate powder
- 1/4 cup almonds blended into fine powder in a high-speed blender

Mix with hands into bite-size balls.

*Vita-Mix® is recommended as the ideal high-speed blender.

Zesty Goji Juice or Jam

Depending on the amount of liquid added, you can make a juice or jam.

- 1/4 cup goji berries, soaked. Keep and use soak water.
- 1/2 tsp. orange zest
- 1/2 tsp. fresh grated ginger
- 1 tsp. raw honey, agave nectar, or 1 pitted date

FOR JAM:

Blend well in blender until pureed.

FOR JUICE:

Add 1 cup coconut water, purified water, or apple juice.

Goji Cream Pudding

> meat of two young coconuts
>
> 2 tbsp. goji berries
>
> 1 tbsp. raw honey
>
> 1/2 cup coconut water
>
> 1 vanilla pod (inside beans scraped out)
>
> 1 pinch Celtic sea salt (finely ground)

Crack open two coconuts. Remove the coconut water. Scrape out all the coconut meat inside. Blend all ingredients in a high-powered blender until smooth and creamy. Sprinkle with raw organic cacao nibs. Refrigerate until well chilled. Enjoy!

Fly High Goji Berry Superfood Bonanza

> 4 cups of your favorite liquid (water, hot or cold tea, coconut water, or any nut milk)
>
> 3 tbsp. goji berries
>
> 3 tbsp. cacao powder
>
> 1 tbsp. cacao nibs
>
> 1 tbsp. maca, red maca, or maca extreme
>
> 1 tsp. goji berry extract powder (optional, but super energizing!)
>
> 1–2 tbsp. sweetener (such as yacon syrup, light or dark agave, or any raw honey)
>
> 1–3 cups frozen, organic berries
>
> 1 tbsp. hempseed
>
> 1 small pinch Celtic sea salt
>
> 1/4 leaf fresh aloe vera gel (optional)

Blend all ingredients in a high-powered blender until smooth.

White Chocolate Orange Goji Berry Fudge!

Recipe by Ginger Robinson

Grind up:

　1/2 cup goji berries (this will be sticky, not a powder)

Blend until smooth:

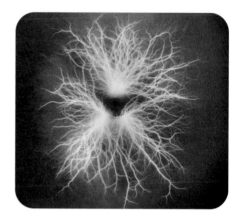

　1/2 cup melted cacao butter

　1/2 cup raw cashews

　1/2 cup agave nectar

Blend in ground gojis.

By hand, mix in whole:

　1/2 cup cacao nibs (optional)

　1/2 cup whole goji berries

　zest from 1 orange

Spread in a glass pie plate (think chocolate almond bark). Chill in the freezer until firm. Enjoy!

Note on Goji Berry Broth

One winter on the Big Island of Hawaii, I was really on a kick for brewing up some fine goji teas. I had been reading about the gelatin content of bone broth, that this was the healing agent attributed to longevity in so many cultures throughout the world. As one can see, the gelling effect fish broths have when put in the fridge is the sign that they have a high gelatin content. The goji insight came when I pulled a very strong goji tea out of the fridge, and it was gelatinized just like fish broth! I had been told that making tea with goji berry was the common practice in Traditional Chinese Medicine, often a base for adding in other herbs, as well as reading about the two-hundred-plus-year-old Taoist Herbalist who drank goji soup every day. Seems that goji is the healing broth of choice for plant people.

—Scott Fraser, superfoodist

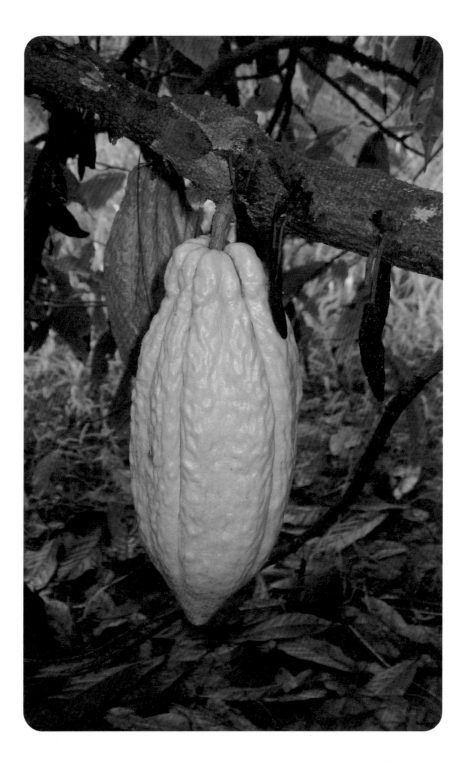

Cacao

Raw Chocolate

Latin Names:

Theobroma cacao

Common Names:

Cacao, cocoa, chocolate, xocolatl (Aztec)

Superfood Type:

Nut

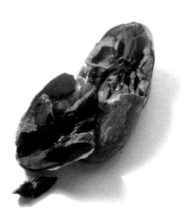

History, Facts, and Legends

There is something about chocolate; there is something in chocolate; there is something we know about chocolate that is beyond touch, taste, and tantalizing sensation. The essence of chocolate is truly indescribable, ineffable, inexpressible.

All chocolate is made from cacao beans (also known as cocoa beans). Cacao is chocolate. All the antioxidant value, mineral benefits, neuro-transmitter rejuvenating properties, and overall health-giving qualities of chocolate are found in original cacao. Chocolate consists of just one ingredient—no sugar, no dairy, no chemicals required—that one ingredient is cacao.

Cacao is the seed (nut) of a fruit of an indigenous American jungle tree. In 1753 Carl Linnaeus, the eighteenth-century Swedish scientist, thought cacao was so important that he named the genus and species of this tree himself: *Theobroma cacao,* or "Cacao, the food of the gods."

Studies on Chocolate

Every study on chocolate is pointing to the same conclusion: there is something in chocolate that is really good for us. That something is the raw cacao bean, the nut that all chocolate is made from. The cacao bean has always been and will always be Nature's number-one weight loss and high-energy food. Cacao beans are probably the best-kept secret in the entire history of food.

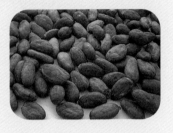

From what I have been able to assess from my own magical mystery cacao tour and visiting cacao growing regions in Central and South America, it appears there was an early, widespread territory of *Theobroma cacao* throughout the north and western portion of Amazonia as well as the Orinoco river basin of Venezuela, along with regions of Central America and Southern Mexico. Over time, various populations of this once heavily forested area were cut off from each other and split into separate ecological niches.

There is no cacao season—chocolate is always in season. The cacao tree flowers and produces fruit all year long. The cauliflori flowers have five petals with pale, lightly scented, mushroom-like growths that grow straight out of the trunk or large branches.

Cacao flowers are rarely visited by bees. They are best pollinated by tiny insects called midges. At least six different types of midges are known to help pollinate cacao. Once pollinated, each flower develops into a pod-fruit. The fruits typically begin as green in color and develop into characteristic red, orange, yellow, blue, or purple varieties. It takes five or six months for each fruit pod to ripen. The fruits usually grow to between seven and eight inches in length. Each fruit contains anywhere from twenty to fifty almond-like seeds, or "beans," surrounded by a sweet, thin pulp. It is these seeds that we call "the food of the gods," or cacao beans—the raw, natural form of chocolate.

Three major species variations of *Theobroma cacao* are currently in wide cultivation around the world: *Criollo, Forastero,* and *Trinitario* (a cross of the other two). *Criollo* is the most highly prized. Many Internet sites and chocolate companies brag about their *Criollo* cacao beans, when in reality they have *Forastero* varieties. *Criollo* varieties are rare, comprising less than 1 percent of the worldwide cacao market.

The cacao fruit is hard-shelled and does not fall to the jungle floor when ripe. In the wild, the ripe cacao fruits are gnawed into by monkeys, birds (macaws, parrots, etc.), bats, and other jungle animals. Typically, some of the seeds fall in the jungle forest and, with good conditions, a new tree is born.

Cacao seeds sprout quite easily, and young trees can bear fruit within three to five years in a proper growing environment. A mature cacao tree will produce about fifty fruits, usually picked two or three times a year. As mentioned, cacao trees bear fruit all year long. Like coconuts and noni, there is no true harvest season. Cacao trees prefer well-drained acidic soils with a high content of organic matter and mushroom mycelium. As long as that type of soil is present, close companion trees do not bother the cacao. Trees and plants such as *annona* trees (cherimoya family), avocado trees, bananas, coconut palms, legume-shade trees, oil palms, rubber trees, and many other tropicals are intercropped with cacao.

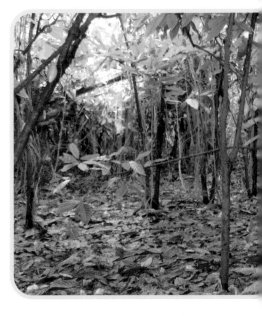

Cacao trees grow best in the shade of larger trees where they are protected from wind and excessive sun. They like to grow inside the latitudes of 20 degrees north and 20 degrees south of the equator. Within this zone, cacao trees can adapt to a large range of tropical conditions (from extremely humid to drier regions), but they must have warm temperatures to thrive (79 degrees Fahrenheit or 21 degrees Celsius is ideal). They love environments

Cacao instead of Gold

Cacao beans were so revered by the Mayans and Aztecs that they used them instead of gold as money!

When political turmoil caused Cortez to return to Spain in 1528, he brought with him precious minerals, agricultural goods and, most likely, cacao beans. Cortez was probably the first to bring chocolate to Europe. The world would never be the same. About the cacao drink, he wrote it was: "The divine drink which builds up resistance and fights fatigue. A cup of this precious drink permits a man to walk for a whole day without food."

where temperatures are above 60 degrees F (16 degrees C). They thrive best with minimal fluctuations of high humidity. All of these factors make cacao a great house or greenhouse plant. You can purchase cacao trees over the Internet for your home or greenhouse. If conditions are just right, in a few years, your cacao trees will actually bear fruit.

When the conquistador Cortez and his henchmen first encountered the Aztecs, the Spaniards were amazed to find a thriving highland metropolis known as Tenochtitlan nestled between the peaks of fifteen mountains, most of them volcanic. At that time, Tenochtitlan (now Mexico City) boasted more than a million residents, making it several times larger than the greatest cities in Europe. Cortez and his crew were confronting a completely unique ecosystem, civilization, and culture. What

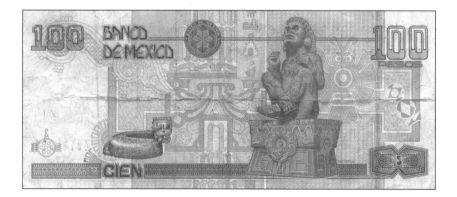

Cacao

Cortez and his men found most shocking was the fact that Emperor Montezuma's royal coffers were overflowing, not with gold, but with cacao beans. Gold was used in the Aztec empire for aesthetic purposes, not for money. The coin of the realm in ancient Mexico was cacao beans. The Spanish chronicler Francisco Cervantes de Salazar mentions that the Emperor's cacao warehouse held more than 40,000 loads, which would mean 960,000,000 beans!

Cacao spread from the royal court of Spain into France, Holland, England, Belgium, and Italy, and eventually across all of Western Europe. It was the Europeans who combined cacao with refined cane sugar; the Native Americans always preferred bitter chocolate. We now know that refined sugar draws minerals out of the body, causes blood sugar disorders, dehydration, and is highly addictive. Sugar, with all its attendant dangers, lowered the medicinal value of the chocolate sold in Europe and altered the spirit of cacao's original healing properties.

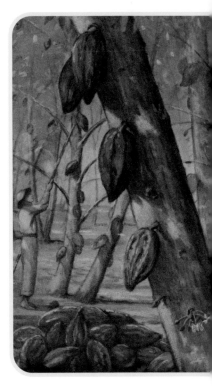

Bioko, a small island near the equator off the coast of west Africa, was the first site of cacao cultivation outside of the Americas. Farmers planted cacao from Venezuela there in 1590 so that the cacao trade could be closer to Europe. This island with its well-drained soil, tropical rain patterns, and warm climate, possesses a perfect climate for cacao. Bioko became the launch point for cacao into Africa. The island is now part of the African nation of Guinea. Today, farmers there produce eight thousand tons of cacao beans each year, accounting for 70 percent of the nation's export wealth.

In 1828, a Dutch chemist named Coenraad Johannes Van Houten patented a process for the manufacture of a new kind of low-fat powdered chocolate. As early as 1815, in his Amsterdam factory, he had been looking for a better method than boiling and skimming to remove most of the cacao butter from chocolate. He eventually developed a very efficient hydraulic press that squeezed the oil out of the cacao. Cacao typically contains around 50 percent cacao oil/butter, but when the cacao was processed through Van Houten's machine, the cacao was reduced to around

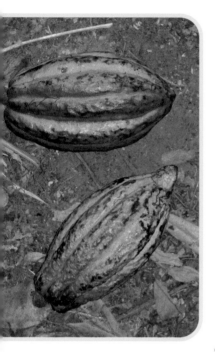

27 percent oil/butter leaving a "cake" that could be pulverized into a fine powder. Van Houten created what would eventually be termed "cocoa or cocoa powder." To cause his cocoa powder to mix well with water, Van Houten treated it with alkaline salts (potassium or sodium carbonates). While this "Dutching," as it came to be known, improved the powder's miscibility (not its solubility) in warm water, it also made the chocolate darker in color and milder in flavor. Van Houten's invention made it possible to develop large-scale manufacturing and distribution of cheap chocolate in powdered and solid forms that millions of people could afford.

The invention of notoriously problematic milk chocolate was due to the collective effort of two men: the Swiss chemist Henri Nestlé (1814–1890) and Swiss chocolate manufacturer Daniel Peter (1836–1919). In 1867, Nestlé discovered a process to powder milk by evaporation. This discovery eventually made Nestlé's business enterprise the largest food corporation in the world. Daniel Peter came up with the idea of using Nestlé's milk powder in a new kind of chocolate. In 1879, the first milk chocolate bar was produced.

The Sacred Heart

More than anything else, cacao supports the heart in a literal, metaphysical, and spiritual sense. The Aztecs often called cacao *yollotl eztli*, which means "heart blood." Cacao supports a healthy cardiovascular system, opens the heart, returns us to our natural state of feeling (instead of

With cacao there is fantastic hope for chocoholics everywhere! You can turn cravings for cooked, processed chocolate into super-nutrition with raw chocolate (raw cacao beans, nibs, butter, powder, and bars).

excessive thinking), and reconnects us via intuition to the mystery of Mother Nature's herbal apothecary.

The mythology surrounding cacao seems to always revolve around regaining the human heart connection to Mother Nature. Consider the following legend from South America:

Khuno, the god of storms, destroyed a village with torrential rain and hail because he was angry at the people for having set fire to the jungle to clear land for their crops. After the storm, the people found a cacao tree. This, they say, is how cacao came into cultivation. Cacao showed these people how to live in harmony with the jungle.

Like all superfoods, chocolate straddles the line between a food and a potent and beneficial medicine.

The raw cacao bean is one of nature's most fantastic superfoods due to its mineral content and wide array of unique properties. Since many of the special properties of cacao are destroyed by cooking, refining, and processing, planet Earth's favorite food is still unknown to most of us. Now we get to reconnect with the power of real chocolate.

Benefits

This raises the possibility that certain food components like cocoa flavonols may be beneficial in increasing brain blood flow and enhancing brain function among older adults or for others in situations where they may be cognitively impaired, such as fatigue or sleep deprivation.

—Ian A. Macdonald, University of Nottingham Medical School, commenting on promising research on cocoa (cacao) and the improvement of mental acuity research.

Cacao Is the Best Natural Food Source of the Following Nutrients

Antioxidants

Cacao contains the highest concentration of antioxidants of any food in the world. These antioxidants include polyphenols, catechins, and epicatechins. By weight, cacao has more antioxidants than red wine, blueberries, açai, pomegranates, and goji berries combined.

Antioxidants protect us from age-related health conditions and illnesses. They shield our DNA from free-radical damage. High antioxidant superfoods like cacao, as a general rule, potentiate the superherbs such as medicinal mushrooms (reishi, cordyceps, chaga, maitake, shiitake, lion's mane, coriolus, etc.), astragalus, pau d'arco, cat's claw, and others.

Magnesium

Cacao seems to be the number one source of magnesium, one of the great alkaline minerals.

Magnesium supports the heart, increases brainpower, causes strong peristalsis (bowel movements), relaxes menstrual cramping, relaxes muscles, increases flexibility, helps build strong bones, and increases alkalinity.

When the body has enough magnesium, veins and arteries breathe a sigh of relief and relax, which lessens resistance and improves the flow of blood, oxygen, and nutrients throughout the body. Studies show that a deficiency of magnesium is not only associated with heart trouble but that immediately following a heart attack, lack of sufficient magnesium promotes free-radical injury to the heart.

Magnesium is the most deficient major mineral on the Standard American Diet (SAD); over 80 percent of North Americans are chronically deficient in magnesium. Cacao has enough magnesium to help reverse deficiencies of this mineral.

Iron

Cacao contains 314 percent of the U.S. RDA (Recommended Daily Allowance) of iron per 1 ounce (28 gram) serving. As is now well known, iron is a critical mineral in nutrition. Iron is part of the oxygen-carrying protein called hemoglobin that keeps our blood healthy and fights back anemia.

Chromium

Chromium is an important trace mineral that helps balance blood sugar. Nearly 80 percent of Americans are deficient in this trace mineral. Cacao contains enough chromium to help reverse deficiencies in this mineral.

Manganese

Cacao is a rich source of manganese, an essential trace mineral. Manganese helps assist iron in the oxygenation of the blood and formation of hemoglobin. Interestingly, manganese is also concentrated in tears.

Zinc

Cacao is an excellent source of zinc, another essential trace mineral. Zinc plays a critical role in the immune system, liver, pancreas, sexual fluids, and skin. Additionally, zinc is involved in thousands of enzymatic reactions throughout the human body. Zinc becomes more bioavailable after

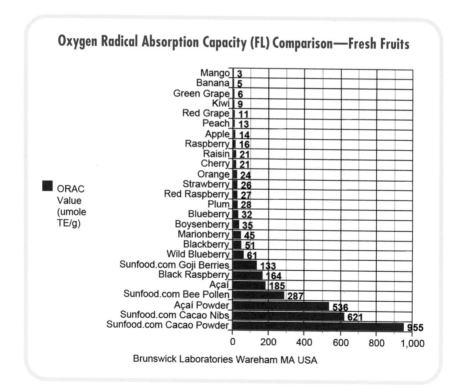

Oxygen Radical Absorption Capacity (FL) Comparison—Fresh Fruits

ORAC Value (umole TE/g)

Fruit	ORAC Value
Mango	3
Banana	5
Green Grape	6
Kiwi	9
Red Grape	11
Peach	13
Apple	14
Raspberry	16
Raisin	21
Cherry	21
Orange	24
Strawberry	26
Red Raspberry	27
Plum	28
Blueberry	32
Boysenberry	35
Marionberry	45
Blackberry	51
Wild Blueberry	61
Sunfood.com Goji Berries	133
Black Raspberry	164
Açaí	185
Sunfood.com Bee Pollen	287
Açaí Powder	536
Sunfood.com Cacao Nibs	621
Sunfood.com Cacao Powder	955

Brunswick Laboratories Wareham MA USA

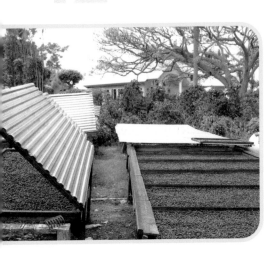

we cleanse and detoxify ourselves of heavy metals.

Copper

Copper is an essential trace mineral. Copper is found naturally as part of the vitamin C complex in plants including cacao. In the human body, copper helps to build healthy blood and strong immunity.

Vitamin C

Ascorbic acid was discovered in 1928 by a scientist from Budapest named Albert Szent-Györgyi. In 1937 he was awarded the Nobel Prize for Physiology and Medicine in recognition of his discoveries concerning the biological oxidation processes, with special reference to vitamin C.

We have Linus Pauling to thank for bringing forth an awareness about the importance and value of vitamin C as both a super-medicine and potentiator of other compounds. Linus Pauling won two Nobel Prizes (Chemistry in 1954 and Peace in 1962).

A one-ounce (28 gram) serving of cacao nibs supplies 21 percent of the U.S. RDA of vitamin C. That's about 44 mg per 100 grams of cacao. This is an extraordinarily high value for a dried nut or seed. Cacao must be raw to contain vitamin C. All cooked and processed chocolate has lost all of its valuable vitamin C.

Omega-6 Fatty Acids

Cacao contains essential omega-6 fatty acids. All cooked and processed chocolate contains rancid omega-6 fatty acids (trans fat) that can cause an inflammatory reaction when one eats cooked chocolate. This is the final arbiter on the matter of raw versus cooked chocolate. Chocolatiers

Cacao is great fun for everyone—especially kids!

cannot escape the fact that once the cacao bean is cooked their product is automatically contaminated with rancid essential fatty acids.

Phenylethylamine (PEA)

Phenylethylamines (PEAs) are a class of compounds found in abundance in cacao. There are different frequencies of phenylethylamines in cacao that are either destroyed or coagulated by roasting cacao beans. Because phenylethylamines are heat-sensitive, they are not present in conventional and organic cooked and processed chocolate.

PEAs are a major class of chemicals that we produce in our bodies when we fall in love. This is likely one of the main reasons why love and chocolate have such a deep connection. PEAs also play a role in increasing focus and alertness.

A greater than 2.2 percent concentration of PEAs and a significant concentration of magnesium appear to be the main natural appetite suppressants found in cacao.

Cacao beans contain no sugar and approximately 50 percent fat depending on variety and growth conditions. A 50 percent fat content is actually low compared to other nuts. There is no evidence to implicate cacao bean consumption with obesity. Cacao is actually one of the great weight-loss foods because within its extraordinary nutrition profile it contains the minerals and PEA molecules that shut off appetite.

Anandamide

Anandamide is a cannabinoid endorphin that the human body naturally produces after exercise. Anandamide has only been found in one plant—cacao. Anandamide is known as the "bliss chemical" because it is released while we are feeling great. Cacao contains enzyme inhibitors that decrease our bodies' ability to breakdown anandamide. This means that when we eat cacao,

> *The ascorbic acid [vitamin C] in foodstuffs is easily destroyed by cooking at high temperatures, especially in the presence of copper and to some extent of other metals....*
>
> *If we lived entirely on raw, fresh plant foods, as our ancestors did some millions of years ago, there would be no need for concern about getting adequate amounts of the essential foods, such as the vitamins.*
>
> —Linus Pauling, *Vitamin C, the Common Cold, and the Flu*

natural anandamide and/or cacao anandamide tend to stick around longer, making us feel good longer.

Tryptophan

Cacao contains significant quantities of the essential amino acid tryptophan, a powerful mood-enhancing nutrient. According to research obtained by cross-referencing data on the Internet, cacao powder consists of somewhere between 0.2–0.5 percent tryptophan.

The presence of tryptophan in the diet is critical for the production of serotonin, our primary neurotransmitter. Once in our bodies, tryptophan reacts with vitamin B6 and vitamin B3 in the presence of magnesium to produce serotonin. Enhanced serotonin function typically diminishes anxiety and literally improves our neurological and physiological "stress-defense shield."

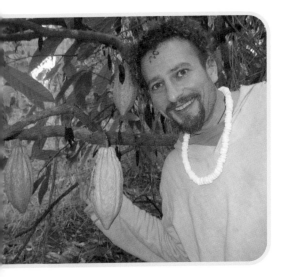

Tryptophan is heat-volatile and susceptible to damage or destruction by cooking. As a result, tryptophan is usually deficient in many cooked-food diets, even if animal protein intake is high. (This may be a large reason why depression is on the rise.) Eating cacao beans raw would thus be an excellent way to obtain dietary tryptophan.

Serotonin

Cacao is rich in the tryptamine serotonin. Serotonin is the primary neurotransmitter in the human body and in nearly all living things. Serotonin is similar in its chemistry to tryptophan, melatonin, and DMT. Serotonin helps us build up our "stress-defense shield." If serotonin levels are high, the world could be collapsing and we would still feel good. If serotonin levels are low, all could be well, but we would still feel like hell.

Fiber

Cacao contains an extraordinary type of soluble fiber. The fiber is so perfect for the human digestive system that cacao can be blended, crushed, and micronized and will still help cleanse the intestines and bulk up bowel movements.

Methylxanthines: Caffeine and Theobromine

Does cacao contain caffeine? Contrary to popular opinion, cacao is a poor source of caffeine. A typical sample of cacao nibs or beans will yield anywhere from zero caffeine to 1,000 parts per million of caffeine (less than 1/20th of the caffeine present in conventional coffee).

Today we know that cacao is one of the richest sources of a peculiar and interesting substance known as theobromine, a close chemical relative and metabolite of caffeine.

Theobromine, like caffeine, and also like the asthma-improving methylxanthine theophylline, belong to the chemical group known as xanthine alkaloids. Chocolate products contain some caffeine, but not nearly enough to explain the attractions, fascinations, addictions, and effects of chocolate.

Cacao usually contains about 1 percent theobromine. Theobromine is an effective antibacterial substance that kills *streptococci mutans* (the primary organism that causes cavities). Theobromine is a chemical relative of caffeine but is not a nervous system stimulant. Theobromine dilates the cardiovascular system, making the heart's job easier. This is

> ## Cacao—Chinese Medicine
>
> Treasures: Yang jing, qui/qi, shen, blood
>
> Atmospheric Energy: subtly cooling (in excess ... heating)
>
> Taste: sweet, bitter, astringent
>
> Organ Association: heart, kidneys, spleen

one of the major reasons why cacao is an important part of a heart-healthy diet.

In February 2008, Dr. Gabriel Cousens discovered in clinical tests of healthy people that cacao does not elevate blood sugar in the same way as a caffeine-containing food or beverage. In fact, Dr. Cousens found that cacao has less of an effect on blood sugar than nearly any other food. Cacao raises blood sugar by only 6 to 10 percent. Foods containing stimulants can raise the blood sugar by more than 30 percent.

Does Cacao Contain Harmful Oxalic Acid?

Cacao contains somewhere between 1,520 and 5,000 parts per million oxalic acid. Is this harmful? When considering more common foods that are much higher in oxalic acid such as spinach, the answer is clearly no. Also, keep in mind that once oxalic acid is cooked it binds with calcium in the body and settles in the kidneys. Another reason to eat raw chocolate.

Here are a few listings of oxalic acid amounts from a table originally published in *Agriculture Handbook No. 8-11, Vegetables and Vegetable Products* in 1984:

Vegetable Oxalic Acid (g/100 g)

Amaranth	1.09
Parsley	1.70
Purslane	1.31
Spinach	0.97

In this table, raw chocolate would rate between 0.15 and 0.50. At the very most, it still has half the oxalic acid content of spinach. Consider how much chocolate people eat versus how much spinach—you may easily decide to eat 100 grams (3.5 oz) of raw spinach in a salad, but try eating 3.5 oz of chocolate in the same amount of time. You'll have more on your mind than oxalic acid.

Cardiovascular Cleansing Compounds

Like goji berries, cacao contains the compounds *N-caffeoyldopamine* and *N-coumaroyldopamine* and their analogs. These compounds significantly suppress an adhesive molecule, *P-selectin,* that glues platelets to white blood cells and blood-vessel walls and increases inflammation. Elevated *P-selectin* levels in the blood have been associated with an elevated danger of cardiovascular clots (thromboses).

What to Look For...

Cacao Product Types

Look for the following raw, organic cacao products:

Cacao beans with the skin
Cacao beans without the skin
Cacao nibs
Cacao with fruit (this still has the dried, sweet cacao fruit on the unfermented bean)
Cacao powder
Cacao butter
Cacao paste

Cacao

Planetary Association: Sun—Center of the Sun
Specific Organ Effect Location: Sacred Heart
Sex: Slightly male
Cosmic lover: Vanilla

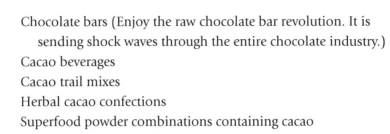

Chocolate bars (Enjoy the raw chocolate bar revolution. It is
   sending shock waves through the entire chocolate industry.)
Cacao beverages
Cacao trail mixes
Herbal cacao confections
Superfood powder combinations containing cacao

[Note: It takes approximately 2^1/$_2$ to 3 pounds of raw cacao nibs/beans to create one pound of raw cacao butter.]

When buying cacao, look for the following to make sure you are getting the highest-quality "bang for the buck":

Low microbe counts: Because of the exceptional quality and standards under which www.sacredchocolate.com's cacao products are processed, any foreign microbe/bacteria activity is virtually nonexistent on the skin and inner nib. This is an extraordinary feat considering that cacao beans come from a moist and juicy fruit grown in the hot jungle. The unique process Sacred Chocolate uses to dry cacao nibs and beans retains the purity, fine aroma, fairly uniform large size, purplish-brown color, easy peeling (of the beans), and nutritional impact that nature intended. Because of the quality of the bean and of the processing, you get to enjoy a rich, raw chocolate flavor and aroma without roasting. Sacred Chocolate takes care to deliver you the finest, cleanest, microbe-free organic cacao beans, nibs, butter, and powder available on the world market. Be aware that poor-quality cacao is also available that has been heated, fumigated, fermented, conventionally grown, and/or may even be dirty (contaminated with dirt as well as bacteria and fungi).

Pleasant and tasty. Great flavor without roasting. Low acidity and no-to-low fermentation.

100 percent raw and certified organic. Purchase Fair Trade or better quality organic cacao to ensure your cacao and chocolate products have not been harvested by slave labor. A Fair Trade certification is not necessarily required to indicate quality or slavery-free cacao yet it is an important standard for conventionally-grown cacao coming from Africa. Sacred Chocolate currently pays cacao farmers nearly four times the Fair Trade standard, and, in cooperation with other companies, is helping to develop an even higher standard of farmer protection.

John Robbins, the author of *Diet for a New America* and *The Food Revolution*, founder of EarthSave International and of the Web site www.foodrevolution.org, has suggested seven things you can do to stop the use of slaves in cacao harvesting in Africa and other nations:

1. Educate yourself further. Good sources of information include:
   Global Exchange (www.globalexchange.org)
   The Child Labor Coalition (www.stopchildlabor.org); Anti-Slavery
     (www.antislavery.org); Unfair Trade (www.unfairtrade.co.uk)
   Fair Trade (www.fairtrade.net)
   Kevin Bales's book *Disposable People* (University of California Press,
     2000) is a thoroughly researched expose of modern-day slavery.

2. Write a letter to the editor or an article in your local newspaper. Blog about these issues on websites. Write to your Congressional representatives and senators.

3. Buy Fair Trade chocolate and/or better-quality cacao products (raw, organic).

Cacao—Ayurveda

Taste: sweet, astringent, bitter
Energy: Cooling (in excess . . . heating)
Post-Digestive Effect: Sweet
Properties and Action on the Tri-Dosha:

Light	Mild laxative
Good for the heart	Drying oil
Dry	

Reduces Vata (in small to moderate quantities)
Reduces Pitta (in small quantities)
Reduces Kapha (in small quantities)
Increases Pitta, Kapha, and Vata (in that order)
  (in excessive quantities)

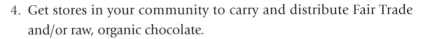

4. Get stores in your community to carry and distribute Fair Trade and/or raw, organic chocolate.

5. Contact the big chocolate companies and ask them to buy Fair Trade cacao. Hershey Foods Corp. can be reached at 100 Crystal A Drive, Hershey, PA 17033; (717) 534-6799; Mars, Inc. can be reached at 6885 Elm Street, McLean, VA 22101; (703) 821-4900. Tell them that you expect something to be done immediately to ensure that cacao imported into the U.S. is not harvested by enslaved children.

6. Support the Fair Trade campaign by joining organizations such as Global Exchange. They can be reached at 2017 Mission Street, #303, San Francisco, California 94110; (415) 255-7296; info@globalexchange.org.

7. Support the anti-slavery movement by joining organizations such as Anti-Slavery International. They can be reached in the U.S. at Suite 312-CIP, 1755 Massachusetts Avenue, NW, Washington, DC 20036-2102. The main office is Anti-Slavery International, Thomas Clarkson House, The Stableyard, Broomgrove Road, London SW9 9TL, England.

How to Use Cacao Products

After eating chocolate you feel godlike, as though you can conquer enemies, lead armies, entice lovers.

—Emily Luchetti, author and pastry chef

Recommended ways to consume chocolate:

1. Purchase raw cacao products (beans, nibs, powder, butter) and blend them into your favorite beverage. One tablespoon of cacao powder per quart works great with any beverage. Blend cacao into coconut water, teas, or coffee. Discover the magic of cacao drinks.

2. Sprinkle raw cacao beans (nibs) on your favorite dessert or treat instead of chocolate chips. Raw cacao beans ARE the original chocolate chips.

3. Eat raw cacao beans with goji berries, hempseed, Incan berries,

almonds, and other trail mix ingredients. Cacao is truly an outrageous snack food!

4. Eat raw cacao beans by themselves. If you are a dark chocolate fan, you will hardly believe the truth about chocolate.

Please read my book *Naked Chocolate* to discover all the subtle nuances of cacao alchemy.

Recommended Daily Intake

Small quantities of cacao per person per day: 1 cacao bean per 17–22 pounds weight.

Moderate quantities of cacao per person per day: 1 cacao bean per 11–17 pounds of body weight.

Excessive quantities of cacao per person per day: 1 cacao bean per 3–9 pounds of body weight.

Example 1: If someone weighs 140 pounds, then a moderate intake of cacao beans would be 8–13 cacao beans.

Example 2: If someone weights 200 pounds, and s/he wanted to guzzle massive amounts of cacao, then an excessive amount of cacao would be 22–66 cacao beans.

Cacao Recipes

Fly High Goji Berry Bonanza

4 cups liquid—water, hot or cold tea, fresh coconut water, or any nut milk

3 tbsp. cacao powder

1 tbsp. cacao nibs

1 tbsp. maca or red maca (you can also add a small amount of maca extreme if you desire)

3 tbsp. goji berries

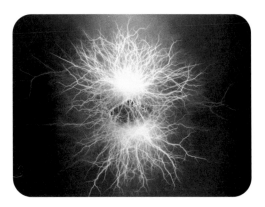

(continued on next page)

1 tsp. goji berry extract powder (optional, but super energizing!)

1–2 tbsp sweetener (we suggest yacon syrup, light or dark agave, or any of our raw honeys)

1–3 cups frozen, organic berries (blueberries, raspberries, and blackberries work well)

1 tbsp. hempseed

1 small pinch Celtic sea salt

1/4–1/2 leaf fresh aloe vera gel (optional)

several drops "Crystal Energy" (optional)

Blend all ingredients in a high-powered blender until smooth.

Oh WOW Cacao—Superfood Greens Booster!

4 cups liquid—water, hot or cold tea, fresh coconut water, or any nut milk

3 tbsp. cacao powder

1 tbsp. maca or red maca (you can also add a small amount of maca extreme if you desire)

1 tbsp. cacao nibs

2 tbsp. coconut butter

1 tbsp. cashews or wild jungle peanuts

1–2 tbsp. sweetener (we suggest yacon syrup, light or dark agave, or raw honey)

1 tbsp. hempseed

1 small pinch Celtic sea salt

1/4–1/2 leaf fresh aloe vera gel (optional)

2 tbsp. green powdered superfoods (select your favorite brand containing superfoods, superherbs, vegetables, grasses, seaweeds, etc.)

1/2–1 tbsp. spirulina

several drops "Crystal Energy" (optional)

Blend all ingredients in a high-powered blender until smooth.

Chocolate Vanilla Bean Dream

- 4 cups liquid—water, hot or cold tea, fresh coconut water, or any nut milk
- 3 tbsp. cacao powder
- 1 tbsp. maca or red maca (you can also add a small amount of maca extreme if you desire)
- 1 tsp. cinnamon
- 1 tbsp. cacao nibs
- 2 tbsp. coconut butter
- 1 tbsp. cashews or wild jungle peanuts
- 1–2 tbsp. sweetener (we suggest yacon syrup, light or dark agave, or raw honey)
- 1 tbsp. hempseed
- 1 small pinch Celtic sea salt
- 1/2 tsp. ginger (optional)
- 1/2–1 tsp. cayenne (optional)
- 1/4–1/2 leaf fresh aloe vera gel
- 1/2 fresh vanilla bean
- 3–5 capsules of medicinal mushroom powders (open capsules and pour powder in)
- several drops "Crystal Energy" (optional)

Blend all ingredients in a high-powered blender until smooth.

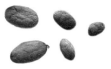

Party Recipes

Cinnamon Rolls

Makes 10 of these gorgeous little bites.

    1 serving dark chocolate sauce (raw cacao beans)
    2–3 pinches ground cinnamon
    1 cup pecans, not soaked
    1 cup medjool dates, pitted

Blend the pecans and the dates together in a food processor to make a dough. Dust some cinnamon onto a clean work surface, and place the dough on it. Sprinkle some more cinnamon on top of the dough and flatten it out, adding more cinnamon if it ever gets sticky.

Once the dough is about 0.2 inches thick, and about 6 x 6 inches square, cut the edges so they are even. Spread the chocolate sauce on top.

Pick up one side of the dough and start to roll to the other side, so you end up with a spiraled log. Cut this log into 0.6 inch-wide rolls and serve.

Chocolate Milk Kick

Serves two, though you may find yourself making more!

    1 pint very cold almond milk
    4 tbsp. chocolate powder (crushed cacao beans or nibs)
    2 tbsp. carob powder
    1 tsp. maca powder
    1 tsp. tocotrienols
    4 tbsp. raw agave nectar
    1/4 tsp. powdered ginseng
    1 tsp. cold-pressed hemp oil
    1 tsp. cold-pressed flax oil

Blend all ingredients together and enjoy immediately before we come over and drink it for you! Simple, fun, and tasteful.

Cacao Kapow

Don't be fooled by the simplicity of this meal, it's one of our best ever recipes! Serves 2, and keeps you up all day.

- 2 oranges
- 14 dried apricots, soaked in water 4 to 6 hours
- 1/2 cup almonds, dry
- 1 heaping tablespoon of raw cacao nibs
- 2 tablespoons of raw cacao powder

Juice the oranges. Blend the orange juice with 10 of the apricots, and put into two glasses.

Blend the remaining apricots with the almonds, cacao nibs, and chocolate powder. Keep it still slightly crunchy. Spoon this on top of the orange and apricot blend.

For an extra treat, top with some agave nectar and some orange zest. Wow!

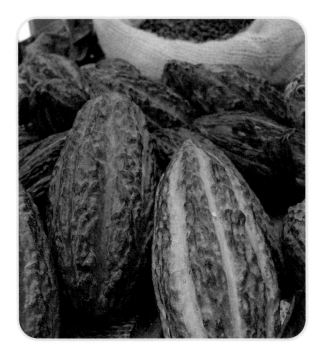

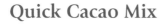
Quick Cacao Mix

3 tbsp. cacao nibs

2 tbsp. hempseed

1/2 tsp. maca or red maca

1 pinch Celtic sea salt

11/2 tbsp. yacon syrup

Combine the first four ingredients in a bowl and mix well, dusting the cacao nibs and hempseed with the maca and Celtic sea salt. Drizzle the yacon syrup over this mixture. Gently fold all ingredients together, so that the cacao nibs and hempseed become evenly coated with yacon syrup. Eat slowly with a spoon. To expand the fun, multiply the above amounts for each person, and share from a bigger bowl! Serves one.

VARIATION 1:

Multiply the amounts of each ingredient by 8

11/2 cups cacao nibs

1 cup hempseed

4 tsp. maca or red maca

1/8 tsp. Celtic sea salt

3/4 cup yacon syrup

Combine first four ingredients in a food processor. Pulse until mixture takes on a thick, sticky consistency. With the food processor on low, pour in a thin stream of yacon syrup until the mixture forms a thick paste (proportions may need to be adjusted). Turn off the processor, and with a dab of coconut oil on each hand, remove the mixture from the bowl in walnut-sized portions. Form into balls, place on a plate, and refrigerate.

Wait at least one hour to enjoy this cool, chocolate snack.

VARIATION 2:

The Traditional Way

Follow the instructions above, but use a large mortar and pestle instead of a food processor. Add $1/2$ teaspoon cayenne pepper with the Celtic sea salt. Grind the ingredients slowly, and channel your love into the best chocolate ever!

Credit: Andrew Rhodes

Chocolate Mint Adorable Smoothie

    3 good scoops frozen almond milk

    2 drops peppermint extract

    1 or 2 scoops Sun Warrior™ rice protein

    1 Sacred Chocolate™ bar (mint variety)

    agave or honey for sweetener (add quantities to your liking)

Break up the chocolate, chop the fruit into small pieces, and place them in the blender. Next add the frozen almond milk and blend until smooth. Serves two.

Chocolate Orange Dream Smoothie

    2 Sacred Chocolate™ bars (Fluffy Citrus variety)

    1 medium/large organic orange

    11/2 cups frozen berries

    1 or 2 good scoops frozen almond milk

    1 or 2 scoops Sun Warrior™ rice protein

    agave or honey for sweetener (add quantities to your liking)

Break up the chocolate, chop the fruit into small pieces, and place them in the blender. Next add the frozen almond milk and blend until smooth. Serves two.

Raw-k Star Superhero Cacao Spheres

Perfect Tour Food

In a food processor, blend the following raw and organic ingredients into a wet cookie-dough consistency. (Be careful, this recipe is rich in calories!)

2 tbsp. coconut cream (butter)

2 tbsp. cashew butter

2–3 tbsp. coconut oil

2–3 tbsp. cacao butter (melted)

1/3 cup cacao beans (peeled) or cacao nibs

1/4 cup goji berries

1/4 cup Incan berries (golden berries)

1/4 cup pumpkin seeds

1/4 cup hempseed

1 tbsp. mesquite (see Glossary of Recipe Ingredients)

5–6 dates, pitted and diced

1 tbsp. cacao powder

1–2 tbsp. of bee pollen

1 tbsp. AFA blue-green algae

1 tbsp. spirulina

1–2 tbsp. acai powder

1 tbsp. maca

1 tbsp. vanilla powder

1 tbsp. reishi mushroom powder (or open up 5–7 reishi mushroom capsules)

1 tsp. powdered cinnamon

1/2 tsp. powdered nutmeg

1/2 tsp. sea salt

1/4 cup wild honey

After you've mixed all the ingredients well, and while the food processor is still turning, add enough spring water to turn the mixture into a big gob of raw cookie dough. Roll into balls and refrigerate or dehydrate.

Choco-Immuno Elixir

Choose one of the following tea recipes below. To create the hot tea base, bring the tea ingredients to just below a boil in 1.5 quarts (1.5 liters) of spring water, then turn off heat and allow to steep covered in the pot for 5 minutes.

TEA RECIPE 1:

 1 handful goji berries

 5 tbsp. pau d'arco (antifungal superherb from the Amazon)

 2 tbsp. cat's claw (antiviral superherb from the Amazon)

 2 tbsp. chanca piedra (anti-nanobacteria superherb from Peru)

 1 whole vanilla bean, sliced into small pieces

TEA RECIPE 2:

 1 tsp. chanca piedra

 1 tsp. pau d'arco

 1 tsp. chuchuhuasi (kidney-adrenal-lower back healing superherb from the Amazon)

 1/2 tsp. cat's claw

Add the strained contents of the hot tea base (above) to a blender already containing:

 1 handful goji berries

 2 tbsp. maca and/or red maca

 1 tbsp. cacao nibs

 1 tbsp. cacao powder

 1 tsp. mesquite powder

 1 tbsp. coconut oil

(continued on next page)

3 tbsp. Manuka, NoniLand™ honey (or other favorite raw honey), yacon syrup, or agave nectar

1 tsp. cinnamon powder

1 tsp. ginger powder

1 tbsp. Sun Warrior™ protein powder (or hempseed protein powder)

contents of 4–6 capsules of powdered medicinal mushroom blend

contents of 2–4 capsules lion's mane medicinal mushrooms

contents of 2–4 capsules cordyceps medicinal mushrooms

contents of 2–4 capsules agaricus blazei medicinal mushrooms

contents of 2–4 capsules reishi medicinal mushrooms

1 pinch cayenne pepper (to taste)

1 tsp. camu camu powder

2–3 drops of orange essential oil or 1/4 tsp. fresh grated orange zest (optional)

1 pinch Celtic sea salt

Blend until completely creamy and frothy. Enjoy the total-body, feel-good experience on your own or with loved ones.

Serves five.

Warning:

Eating cacao may cause you to have THE BEST DAY EVER!

For further information on raw chocolate read *Naked Chocolate* by David Wolfe and Shazzie. Filled with in-depth information and over sixty mouthwatering recipes, *Naked Chocolate* is the product of years of research into superfood nutrition and the phenomenal and enlightening power of cacao.

Up-Your-Crunch Bar

Recipe by Ginger Robinson

Your friends won't believe it when you tell them that you made this at home. Same texture, chewiness—everything—as those chemicalized, dairy-contaminated chocolate bars, only this tastes WAY better! It's amazing!

Combine equal parts:

Agave nectar

Cacao butter

Raw cashews

Add:

1 big handful white mulberries

1 tsp. ho shou wu powder

1 tbsp. maca powder

1–2 tbsp. lucuma powder

Melt the cacao butter in a measuring cup in the dehydrator, add to blender with agave, and cashews. Blend till smooth. Stir in a big handful of dried mulberries by hand and then pour the mix into molds. Set in freezer awhile to harden them up. Thin slice into chocolate bars and have The Best Day Ever!

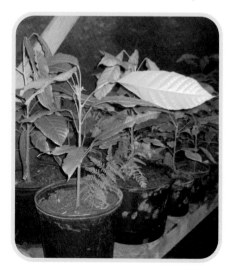

$18,000 Cacao Smoothie

Recipe by Len Foley

Combine base ingredients in a blender:

    1 cup warm gynostemma herbal tea

    1 tbsp. raw virgin coconut oil

    1 tbsp. raw Manuka or NoniLand™ honey

    1 pinch Celtic sea salt

    2 droppersful of liquid Vanilla Creme stevia

Mix on low, then add:

    1 tbsp. hempseed

    1 tbsp. black sesame seeds

Mix on high until smooth, then add:

    Coconut water or raw almond milk or other nut milk
        (up to 3/4 of the mixer)

Add other ingredients:

    5 drops super deer antler

    1 dropperful of liquid zeolites

    4 droppersful of super ionic or angstrom minerals (optional)

    1/2 tsp. ho shou wu powder

    1/8 tsp. eucommia bark powder

    1/2 tsp. maca powder

    1 tbsp. mesquite powder

    1 tbsp. Sun Warrior™ protein powder (or hempseed protein powder)

    11/2–2 tbsp. raw cacao powder

    1 tbsp. Irish sea moss (clean it, must soak 2–3 days, change water
        each day)

    4 caps reishi mushroom

    1/8 tsp. Pure Radiance C® powder

    1/2 tsp. blue-green algae powder

    3 caps blue mangosteen

1/8 tsp. cordyceps mushroom powder

dash of cinnamon powder

1 tbsp. pure pumpkin seed oil

4 caps cistanche powder

2 tbsp. tocotrienols

1 tbsp. bee pollen

Mix on low, then add ice to taste. Continue to mix on low, or a bit higher if necessary, till blended frothy smooth.

"Blend Your Way to Cacao Heaven" Shake

12 oz. spring water or healing tea (suggested combinations: horsetail/oatstraw/nettle or cat's claw/pau d'arco/ho shou wu/reishi)

1/2 inner gel (not skin) from one aloe vera leaf

1–2 tbsp. raw honey (you can also use yacon syrup and/or agave syrup)

1–3 tsp. bee pollen

1 tbsp. coconut oil

1 tbsp. carob powder

1–2 tbsp. mesquite powder

1–2 tbsp. maca powder (also try red maca)

1 tbsp. Sun Warrior™ protein powder (or hempseed protein)

1 tbsp. tocotrienols

2 tbsp. hempseed

1/2–1 tbsp. cold-pressed hempseed oil

2–3 Brazil nuts

2 tbsp. cacao nibs

2 tbsp. cacao powder

1/2 tsp. cacao butter

1–2 tbsp. green powdered superfoods (select your favorite brand containing superfoods, superherbs, vegetables, grasses, seaweeds, etc.)

(continued on next page)

1/4 tsp. blue-green algae powder (try also E3Live™ Flakes or Crystal Manna)

1 tbsp. spirulina

1 pinch Himalayan or Celtic sea salt

1/4 tsp. cinnamon powder

1/4 tsp. chili powder (or more if you like it HOT!)

Combine all ingredients in a high-speed blender and savor the ecstasy of superfood heaven!

Blackie's Chewies

This is like a brownie, only darker and much richer. You can't eat many of these in one go, unless you're a complete raw chocoholic!

4 cups of black mission figs, soaked 1 hour in spring water

1 cup black tahini

1/2 cup raw chocolate powder

1 cup goji berries, soaked 1 hour in spring water

1 tsp. fresh mint leaves

1 tbsp. golden flaxseeds

1–2 tsp. ho shou wu powder

1 tbsp. spirulina

1 pinch Celtic sea salt

Finely grind the flaxseeds in a coffee mill or blender. Put all the ingredients into a food processor and process until fine and doughlike. If the mixture doesn't stick together, slowly add some goji berry soak water while blending.

Knead the dough until you've put lots of love into it, and place it onto a Teflex sheet. Spread it out until it's about 1 inch thick, and square the edges off. Cut into little squares. If you fancy, place half a cherry on top of each square.

Dehydrate for about 4 hours, then turn the squares onto the dehydrator tray without a Teflex sheet and dehydrate for 6 more hours.

¡Olé Mole! Chocolate Tortillas

These are slightly spicy, slightly chocolaty, and oh-so versatile. We stuff them with raw nut/seed pates, avocado, salad, or salsa. Serve them with guacamole, sunflower sprouts, and slices of lime on a bed of spring onions. Makes 6 tortillas.

corn, freshly stripped from 2 raw cobs

1/2 cup dry golden flaxseeds

1/4 avocado

1/2 cup sunflower seeds, dry

4 spring onions

2 cloves garlic

1/4 tsp. Celtic sea salt

1 tsp. cumin powder

1/2 tsp. cayenne powder

1 tbsp. paprika

1 tbsp. raw chocolate powder

2 squeezes lime juice

Ground the flaxseeds into a fine powder using a spice mill. Finely chop the garlic. Chop the spring onions. Add all the ingredients to the food processor and blend until smooth. The dough should be thick and sticky.

Place six equal amounts on a Teflex sheets, flatten out into circles, and dehydrate for about four hours. Turn the tortillas over, remove the Teflex sheets so air can circulate more, and dehydrate for another one or two hours.

Special Note on Allergies

A recent study showed that only one out of five hundred people who thought they were allergic to chocolate actually tested positive. Allergies to chocolate are quite rare. It is typically the case that the person is in fact allergic to milk and dairy products. Some people can be allergic to cooked and processed chocolate but are not allergic to cacao.

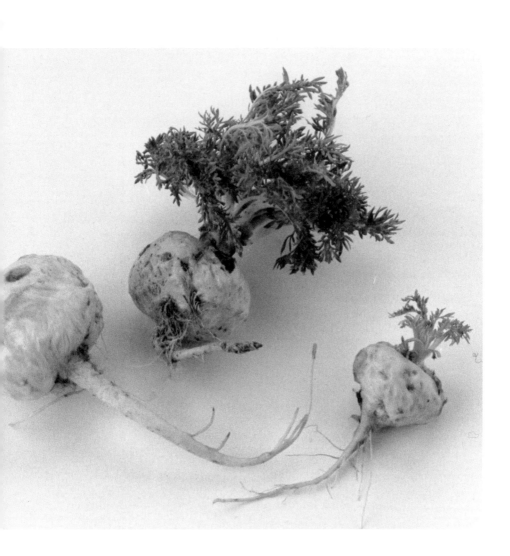

Maca
Andes Aphrodisiac

Latin Names:

Lepidium meyenii, Lepidium peruvianum

Common Names:

Maca, maca root, Peruvian ginseng

Superfood Type:

Root

History, Facts, and Legends

According to archeological evidence, maca has been cultivated and grown high in the Peruvian Andes of South America for approximately 2,600 years.

In her book *Maca: Adaptogen and Hormonal Regulator,* Beth M. Ley, PhD, says that maca was domesticated by the Pumpush, a fierce warrior tribe that migrated into the Andes from the Amazon jungle. Later, the Yaro peoples arrived in the Andean highlands and cultivated immense fields of maca. Eventually, the Incan empire conquered the maca-growing regions of the Andes. Legend has it that during the height of the Incan empire Incan warriors would consume maca before entering into battle to make them fiercely strong, but after conquering a city the Incan soldiers were prohibited from using maca, to protect the women from the excessive sexual desires of the men.

Today the Quechua people, descendants of the Incans, continue to grow this superfood at its natural altitude of 9,000–10,000 feet (2,700–3,000 meters) above sea level and as high as 14,000 feet (4,300 meters), making maca the highest-altitude crop on Earth.

Maca is a member of the cruciferous family of plants that includes broccoli, cabbage, cauliflower, kale, turnips, and radishes.

Maca is grown for its root, which resembles that of the radish, and is off-white, yellow, purple, or yellow in color. Sometimes purple bands streak through the root. Below ground, maca is slightly larger on average than a radish, with a typical diameter of two to three inches. Above ground, maca is quite a bit smaller than its relatives. It produces leaves that grow close to the ground and the plant produces a small, off-white, four-petal flower typical of members of the cruciferous family. Like other cruciferous vegetables and unlike most tuberous plants, maca is propagated by seed instead of by root. Although it is a perennial, it is grown as an annual. Seven to nine months after planting, maca is harvested.

The area where maca is found, high in the Andes, is a barren, treeless, inhospitable region of intense sunlight, turbulent winds, and radical fluctuations in temperature. Daily temperature fluctuations are so great that at sunset temperatures may plummet from a beautiful 64 degrees (18°C) down to 14 degrees Fahrenheit (–10°C) freezing conditions. Because of this, maca has one of the highest frost tolerances among native cultivated species. The character and properties of maca have been developed by

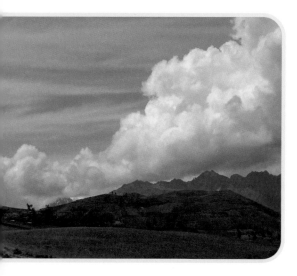

the extreme conditions under which it grows, which makes maca an excellent superfood choice for individuals living in cold climates, at high altitudes, and/or with extreme adventure lifestyles.

Maca has been used medicinally for centuries in South America to enhance fertility in humans and animals. As traditional Andean shamans *(pacos)* state: "When maca is consumed the spirits are close. Maca draws in spirits to be birthed." Soon after the Spanish conquest, the Spanish found that they and their livestock were faring poorly in the barren Andean highlands. The local natives recommended the Spanish eat maca and feed their animals maca. So remarkable were the results that Spanish chroniclers gave in-depth reports. Apparently, some of the first written Spanish records from the Andes are treatises on maca.

Maca was so revered in pre- and post-Spanish conquest times that it was used as currency. Maca was sent to Cusco as tribute to the Incan rulers when they conquered the maca-growing regions. According to Dr. Ley, in 1549 the colonial Spanish government received 15,000 to 18,000 pounds of maca as tribute. Colonial records, now two hundred years old, indicate that payments of roughly nine tons of maca were demanded from the Junin area of the Andes alone for the payment of colonial taxes.

Even today, for many indigenous inhabitants of the Andes, maca is still one of the most vital and valuable of all commodities.

Once harvested, the maca root was traditionally dried, powdered, or cooked. Once dried and/or powdered, it was either eaten or put into sacs and traded for other commodities. Oftentimes cacao nibs and beans (raw chocolate) were traded for maca. Maca and cacao have a unique affinity and history that becomes evident when one eats them together.

In the twentieth century, knowledge about maca nearly died out. In 1979 the Peruvian Department of Agriculture found only seventy acres of maca under cultivation in their country.

There is no doubt that maca has been revivified by one of Peru's leading biologists, Gloria Chacon de Popovici, PhD. Dr. Chacon first published her studies on maca's ability to increase fertility in animals in 1961 and has continued as maca's champion ever since. Her continuing research has demonstrated that maca increases fertility in rats, dogs, guinea pigs, rams, cows, and humans. This research has since been replicated by numerous researchers worldwide.

Maca has not only been a favorite superfood of the Peruvian Quechua people, it has also been enjoyed by raw foodists, vegetarians, adventurers, extreme athletes, dessert chefs, and food alchemists. Now, maca is finally available to individuals across the world.

The renowned effects of maca are creating market demand in Japan, Europe, and North America. With maca cultivation on the increase and a number of Peruvian government experts and agencies actively promoting maca agriculture and development, maca is poised to become a major botanical product on the international superfood and herbal scene.

Benefits

As we've seen, maca's reputation as a powerful strength and stamina enhancer as well as libido-enhancing superfood stretches back into history.

Maca, like the goji berry, reishi mushroom, asparagus root, rhodiola, ginseng, AFA algae, and other superfoods and superherbs, is a powerful adaptogen, which means it has the ability to balance and stabilize the body's glandular-hormonal system, nervous system, cardiovascular system, and musculature.

In 1947, Russian scientist Nikolai Lazarev first defined an adaptogen as a nutritive substance that counters adverse physical, chemical, or biological sources of stress by raising nonspecific resistance, allowing the organism to "adapt" to stressful circumstances.

In 1968, Israel I. Brekhman, PhD, and I. V. Dardymov defined an adaptogen as follows:

1. An adaptogen is nontoxic to the recipient.

2. An adaptogen produces a nonspecific response in the body—an increase in the power of resistance against multiple stressors including physical, chemical, or biological agents.

3. An adaptogen has a normalizing influence on physiology, irrespective of the direction of change from physiological norms caused by the stressor.

Essentially, adaptogens are nontoxic, produce an adaptive response to stress, and improve homeostasis in the body.

According to research, maca as an adaptogenic superfood increases energy, endurance, oxygen in the blood, physical strength, neurotransmitter production, and libido. It supports the endocrine system, the adrenals, and the thyroid, typically improves one's mood, and helps support healthy hormone production.

Consider that maca is known to improve the following conditions:

Anemia
Chronic fatigue
Depression
Infertility and sterility in humans and livestock
Lack of libido
Malnutrition
Menopausal symptoms
Menstrual discomfort and disorders
Poor memory
Stomach cancer
Stress tension
Tuberculosis

Dried maca powder contains approximately 59 percent carbohydrates, 8.5 percent fiber, and slightly more than 10 percent protein. The protein in dried maca powder contains twenty amino acids and seven essential amino acids. Compared to another local Andean root, the potato, maca contains five times more protein and four times more fiber. Although maca is not a complete protein, it is such a great source of hormone precursors and amino acids that it provides many of the same effects created by a high-protein diet.

Maca has a higher lipid (fat) content than other root crops (2.2 percent), of which linolenic acid, palmitic acid, and oleic acid are the primary fatty acids, respectively, and is also a rich source of immune-enhancing sterols, including sitosterol, campesterol, ergosterol, brassicasterol, and ergostadienol. Maca contains biologically active aromatic isothiocyanates, especially p-methoxybenzyl isothiocyanate, which have reputed aphrodisiac properties. Maca is rich in calcium, magnesium, phosphorous, potassium, sulfur, sodium, and iron and contains trace minerals including zinc, iodine, copper, selenium, bismuth, manganese, tin, and silicon. It is also rich in vitamins B1, B2, C, and E.

Women with menstrual irregularities using maca have experienced greater consistency, while women with hot flashes, mood swings, and most associated perimenopause and menopause symptoms have diminished dramatically using maca.

—Beth M. Ley, PhD,
Maca: Adaptogen and Hormonal Regulator

Oxygen and Energy

Maca is known to help us effectively deal with stresses of all types. Because maca increases blood oxygen content it helps to alleviate the environmental stress of altitude sickness (the volume of oxygen at 18,000 feet elevation is typically half of what it is at sea level). When used along with coca tea, nearly all symptoms of altitude sickness can be alleviated in less than an hour.

As an adaptogen, maca can provide more energy if it is needed, but if it is not, it will not overstimulate. According to most studies, adaptogens also boost immunity and increase the body's overall vitality by 10 to 15 percent. Rather than addressing a specific symptom, adaptogens improve the overall adaptability of the whole body to challenging situations and stress.

Endocrine System

Peruvian biologist Gloria Chacon de Popovici, PhD, suggests that maca acts on the hypothalamus and pituitary glands as well as the adrenals. She has theorized that by activating these endocrine glands maca is able to increase energy, vitality, and libido. Other researchers indicate that the effect of maca may be more basic and that when the body is well nourished, libido rises, and depression lowers. Maca's nutrient value could explain some, but not all, of these purported actions.

Dr. Chacon is probably closer to the truth in her scientific reasoning. As Chacon describes, maca works on the master gland of the brain, the hypothalamus. The hypothalamus is generally considered the sex-hormone center of the brain. From the hypothalamus derivative effects occur "downstream" in the way the pituitary gland is stimulated to secrete luteinizing hormone and follicle-stimulating hormone, and the way that the adrenal glands and gonads are stimulated to secrete testosterone, progesterone, and DHEA.

The proper functioning of the endocrine system is deeply correlated with the proper functioning of the immune system. If any part of the endocrine system is out of balance (for example, the adrenals are exhausted), one becomes susceptible to immune system challenges.

In addition, we now know that as we age, the hormone content of our blood, organs, and tissues decreases. Individuals who naturally have a high production of progesterone and/or testosterone are known to stay younger longer. Traditional Western medicine hormone replacement therapies are swiftly converting to more sustainable, reasonable, and intelligent "bio-identical" hormone replacement approaches. However, before we reach for any supplemental hormones, we should first do our best to increase our hormone production with natural superfoods, herbs, and supplements; these include maca and coconut products (wild coconut water and flesh as well as coconut oil and pregnenolone).

Unlike soy products, cohoshes, Mexican wild yams, and flaxseeds, maca is free of plant hormones (such as phytoestrogens and isoflavones).

Aphrodisiac Qualities

We all hear rumors about various products like maca. But using this Peruvian root myself, I personally experienced a significant improvement in erectile tissue response. I call it nature's answer to Viagra. What I see in maca is a means of normalizing our steroid hormones like testosterone, progesterone, and estrogen. Therefore it has the facility to forestall the

Maca has a high nutritional value providing macro and micro nutrients, including traces of 31 different minerals, to support the cellular structures and functioning in the body. Maca can optimize function as it optimizes and balances on a cellular level.

— Dr. Gloria Chacon de Popovici, Biological Sciences, Mayor de San Marcos National University, Lima, Peru

hormonal changes of aging. It acts on men to restore them to a healthy
functional status in which they experience a more active libido.

—Garry F. Gordon, former president of the American College for
Advancement in Medicine

Maca's actions on sexual function are better researched than its effects on
mood and memory. Dr. Gloria Chacon initially demonstrated in her
research that when rats were given maca powder, the male rats had increased
sperm counts and motility rates and the female rats showed multiple egg
follicle maturations. These effects were measurable within seventy-two
hours of feeding the rats maca. Later came studies of guinea pigs, rams,
and cows, each of which corroborated maca's libido-enhancing effects.
For example, maca significantly increased ram semen volume and sperm
count. Researchers such as Dr. Chacon consider plant sterols, isothiocyanates, macamides, and glucosinolates to be maca's active libido- and
fertility-enhancing constituents because when isolated and fed to animals,
these substances demonstrated aphrodisiac qualities.

Maca is one of the greatest superfoods not only because of its caliber
of nutrients, amino acids, and fatty acids, but also because it helps to
increase fertility, so if you are having trouble conceiving a child, maca is
a great superfood to add to your diet. After pregnancy, maca also helps
women to produce more breast milk.

Thyroid Support

Over the years I have had numerous individuals report to me that the regular use of maca either decreased or completely eliminated their thyroid
problems. I have even seen lab reports where medical lab data indicated
that the person should have thyroid problems, but that person did not
because they were taking maca. This indicates an indirect effect that alters
the endocrine system while improving thyroid health without directly
changing the chemistry of the thyroid in a way we know how to test for
at this time.

What to Look For ...

Maca Product Types

Only select reputable, organic brands of maca root—not other parts of the plant. There are no "original" or "true" species of maca, so beware of dubious claims. Below is a list of maca products to look for on the Internet or in your health food store or supplement shop.

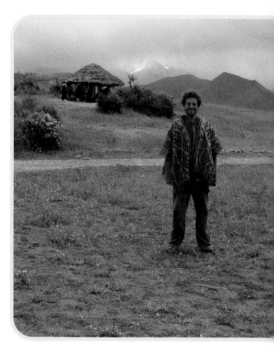

Dried, powdered maca root

Encapsulated, dried, powdered maca root (excellent for traveling)

Red maca

Black maca

Yellow maca

Dried, powdered maca extracts (e.g. Maca Extreme)

Roasted maca

Liquid, alcohol-based maca concentrates

Dried, powdered superfood formulas containing maca as one ingredient

Maca chocolate bars, chocolate brittles, and energy bars

How to Use Maca

Since maca is a superfood, it can be used in greater quantities than other medicinal herbs. It can also be used over a long period of time with no harmful side effects. Maca is a warming food, and therefore is better suited for use in cooler weather and colder climates.

Maca is generally purchased as a dried, raw, organic root powder. You may use a tablespoon or more of this powder in smoothies, teas, nut milks, coffee, or just about any natural beverage you can think of.

As previously mentioned, maca has an unusual relationship with cacao. Mix maca into all your favorite raw chocolate treats and experience real culinary magic.

Maca may also be added to homemade desserts, sweet treats, salads, salad dressings, jams, broths, soups, and puddings.

Maca has a slightly malted flavor and other flavor notes that are sweet and decorated with butterscotch overtones. It also has some minor taste qualities reminiscent of other cruciferous vegetables such as the radish; these qualities add some mild, subtle, spicy elements.

Maca powder is a great emulsifier. It can be used to draw fats/oils together with starches/sugars in a beverage, dessert, or recipe. For example, if one makes a drink containing agave nectar and cacao nibs, maca may be used to draw these two foods smoothly together and create a beautiful, rounded flavor. Another example would be a raw fruit pie with a nutty crust containing figs or dates. If one makes the crust with maca, the nuts and figs or dates will be drawn together for a more wholesome and complete flavor.

A minimum of 0.35 ounces (10 grams per day, or one heaping tablespoon) of the dried root is required for you to notice any real benefit with 0.7 ounces (20 grams per day, or two heaping tablespoons) being the recommended amount. You can increase this considerably if you so desire. It is recommended that you take a week off during every month of consistent use. Sometimes the irregular use of superfoods and superherbs can actually enhance their efficacy.

Can I eat too much maca?

Yes, of course—as with anything in extreme quantities. Maca is a powerful superfood/food/herb and should be consumed with respect, especially by beginners. The first time I ever served maca to one of my best friends, we were in Miami doing a book tour. We kept visiting a favorite juice bar where they served gallons of coconut milk. I had several kilos of maca with me. I asked my friend how many scoops of maca he would like in his coconut milk. He'd never had it before, and said "ten." After consuming ten scoops of maca for his first time ever, it knocked him out. He took more maca than his body could handle because he had never had it before. What was supposed to be a night on the town turned into an early evening.

In toxicity studies conducted in the United States and Peru, maca showed no toxicity and no adverse pharmacological effects. In animal studies, the more maca animals consumed, the stronger and more sexually active they became. In spite of these results, moderation is still advised at least until one is adapted to taking maca.

Can I combine maca with other hormonal types of supplements and herbs?

Yes. Maca can be combined with pregnenolone, DHEA, DIM, black cohosh, wild yam, nettle root, passion flower, etc. with positive effects.

Can maca be used to improve prostate health?

Yes. For men wishing to regain their prostate health and sexual vigor, maca may be mixed or taken with diindolylmethane (DIM). DIM is a compound found in cruciferous vegetables such as a broccoli, kale, and Brussels sprouts that helps regulate hormone balance and cell behavior. DIM is one of the most effective phytonutrients in the prevention and treatment of breast, prostate, colon, and pancreatic cancers.

Studies on the use of DIM in men indicates that it promotes healthy cell formation in the prostate gland. Various research studies have shown that DIM can help reduce the conversion of testosterone into estrogen. An increase in testosterone to estrogen ratio is associated with a healthy prostate gland. Scientific research also shows DIM increases the level of good estrogens (2-hydroxyestrogen) while reducing the level of bad estrogens (16-hydroxyestrogen). Nettle root may also be effectively added to this formula.

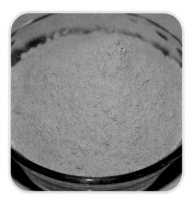

Maca Recipes

Sweet Guaca-Maca Collard Wraps

3 avocados

3 tsp. maca

1/2 tbsp. Celtic sea salt or Himalayan salt

1 tbsp. raw honey

juice of 1 lime

11/2 tsp. spirulina

1 cup sprouted sunflower seeds

1–2 tbsp. raw sesame tahini

Put all ingredients in a bowl and mash or blend in a blender to a creamy consistency. Stuff into collard greens and wrap it up! For an extra kick, add cacao nibs to the guaca-maca!

Maca Extreme Recipes

All the recipes below have a minimum measurement of maca, representing a very light flavor of maca. Use a higher dosage for a stronger flavor.

These recipes use Maca Extreme for several reasons:

- The taste may be easier to integrate into balancing flavors
- It is a higher-quality product due to being dried at lower temperatures
- The absence of fiber in this product allows a higher concentration of certain medicinal properties to be absorbed
- Lastly, depending on when in their cycle certain cruciferous vegetables are harvested, they absorb pollutants, especially of the aldehyde family, from the air, which is great for the environment but not so great for the body, so we have found that when these vegetables have their fiber removed (as is the case with Maca Extreme), the aldehyde concentration is mostly removed as well.

Extreme Warrior Maca Smoothie

    4 cups hemp milk

    1 scoop Sun Warrior™ barley (activated barley)

    1 scoop Sun Warrior™ Natural protein powder (rice protein)

    1 handful goji berries

    1 tbsp. coconut oil

    1 tbsp. Maca Extreme

    1 tbsp. bee pollen

    2 tbsp. raw honey

Blend well. You can also add an also add some cinnamon, vanilla bean, and chocolate powder!

Maca Thai Dressing

Recipe by Kimberly Reschke

    1/2 cup coconut cream or coconut meat

    juice of 1 lime

    2 tsp. raw honey

    1/2 cup hemp oil

    1/2 cup spring water

    1/2–4 tbsp. Maca Extreme

    1 tbsp. basil

    1/2 tbsp. hot chilies

    salt to taste (use Celtic, Himalayan, or your favorite salt)

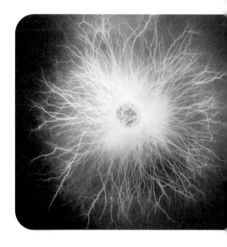

Mix in blender until smooth and it is ready to devour! Use as a salad dressing or with noodle dishes. Pour over cucumber or kelp noodles. Serves 2.

Maca Onion Bread

Recipe by Kimberly Reschke

    6 large onions peeled

    11/2 cups golden flaxseeds, freshly ground

    11/2 cups hempseed nuts, freshly ground

    1 cup Nama Shoyu soy sauce

    2/3 cup olive oil

    2–10 tbsp. Maca Extreme

Toss peeled onions, freshly ground seeds, liquids, and maca into a food processor, blending to even consistency.

Spread about 2 cups of the mixture on a dehydrator tray lined with a Teflex sheet. Repeat to fill four trays. Dehydrate at 110 degrees F for approximately 12 hours, flipping over and peeling off Teflex sheet and dehydrating until ready, usually 4 to 6 more hours.

Enjoy as is, with avocado and tomato for a sandwich, or as a base for raw pizza. A great way to get a healthy, delicious amount of long-chain sugars from onions!

Maca Vanilla Ice Cream

Recipe by Kimberly Reschke

    11/2 cups cool processed raw cashews

    1/2 cup coconut cream or coconut meat

    1/2 cup lucuma powder

    1/2 cup raw honey

    1/2 tbsp. raw vanilla powder or 2 scraped insides of vanilla beans

    11/2 tbsp. psyllium hulls (essential for creating a soft ice cream that can be scooped)

    1/2 cup spring water, or more to allow blending to thick consistency

    1–6 tbsp. Maca Extreme

    salt to taste

Mix the above ingredients into a smooth consistency, pour the mixture into a bowl, and place in the freezer until set. This recipe serves 6.

For an extra-delicious addition, after the ice cream has set for approximately two hours, swirl in the following ingredients to create a hard fudge in creamy vanilla. Warning: it might make you devour the whole bowl in one day!

- 1/2 cup coconut oil warmed to liquid consistency (easy in a dehydrator below 115 degrees)
- 1/4 cup cacao butter warmed to liquid consistency
- 2 tbsp. raw honey
- 1/2 cup cacao powder

White Goddess Chocolate—Jungle Maca Style!

Recipe by Kimberly Reschke

- 2 cups cacao butter (melted on a stove via the double-boiler method or in the dehydrator)
- 11/2 cups coconut cream (sometimes called coconut butter, it contains the fiber)
- 1/2–1 cup raw honey, depending on how sweet you are!
- 3/4 cup jungle peanut butter or ground jungle peanuts
- 1/4 cup lucuma powder
- 11/2–5 tbsp. Maca Extreme
- 1 tbsp. raw vanilla powder or 2 scraped vanilla beans

In a food processor, combine the melted cacao butter with the remaining ingredients. Pour into a pie plate or individual chocolate molds and allow to set in the fridge or freezer. A nice mellow chocolate for kids and adults!

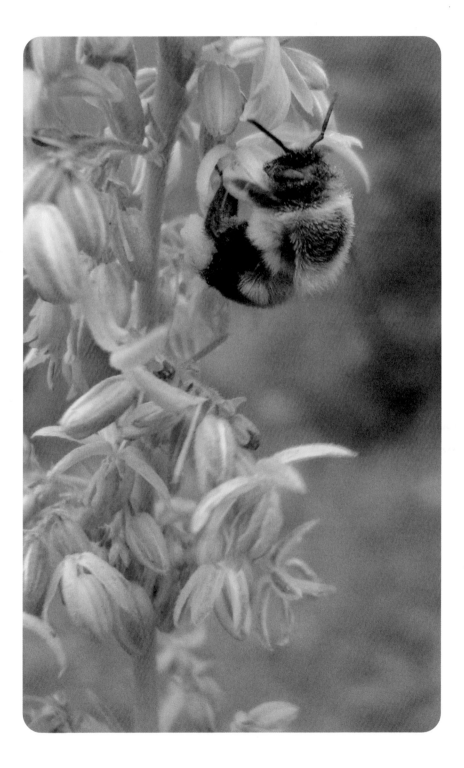

Bee Products
The Original Superfoods

Latin Names:

Honeybees:

Apis mellifera spp.

Apis dorsata

Common Names:

Honey, *miel* (Spanish)

Pollen

Propolis

Royal jelly

Superfood Type:

Honey

Pollen

Royal jelly

Propolis

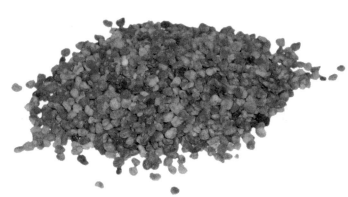

History, Facts, and Legends

No bees, no honey; no work, no money.

The history, legends, and mythology surrounding bees and bee products are so grand that they could fill volumes of books. The only food that comes close to bee products in overall richness of history and legend is chocolate (cacao).

Scientists and archeologists have discovered caves in river valleys of Southern France and Northern Spain that are abundant with paintings and etchings depicting human life in a prehistoric era. Most of the paintings represent large game animals such as deer and bison. One painting found in a cave near Valencia, Spain portrays two men stealing honey from a beehive. The men are balanced on a handmade ladder leaning against a rocky hillside. One of the men is removing the honeycomb from the hive and fighting off an angry swarm of bees as the other man waits below

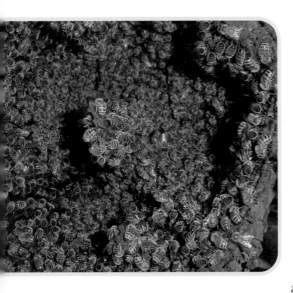

for the honeycomb to be passed down. The bees are depicted many times their normal size to explain and emphasize the events taking place.

Ancient Egypt is where our present-day beekeeping sciences began. The Egyptians were among the first peoples on Earth to keep bees, as recorded in temple wall carvings, and in hieroglyphics on papyri scrolls. Symbols of the bee and beehive appear everywhere throughout Egypt. The symbols are found in jewelry, inscribed on temple walls and tombs, woven into fabrics, carved on the famous Rosetta Stone, and next to the signature of the pharaoh on official documents. The Egyptians offered honey and bee pollen to the gods. Bees and bee products were featured in almost every ritual.

Honey products were also broadly used in Greco-Roman civilization. In both the *Iliad* and *Odyssey,* Homer repeatedly refers to honey and pollen. The famous ancient Greek vegetarian Pythagoras enjoyed honey daily, as did his students. Honey and honey water featured prominently in the ancient Olympic games of Greece; they were used as food and beverage, and for body and skin care during the games. The famous Roman writer Pliny the Elder described a village in the Apennine Mountains near the River Po where the majority of people lived to over one hundred years old due to their consumption of honey and pollen. Pliny's *Natural History* contains a book almost entirely devoted to bees and beehives:

> Book 11: Insects—Bees, hives, the sources of honey, the organization of bees, honeycombs, drones, queen bees, portents provided by bees, bee-stings, the silk-moth, silk production, comparative zoology, and taxonomy: eyes, heart, anthropoid apes, bad breath of animals.

During ancient times the British Isles were known as "The Honey Isle of Beli" for the large quantities of honey they produced. Long after the fall of Rome, honey was used throughout Europe in religious ceremonies, as a medium for barter and exchange, and to pay taxes.

In Arabia, Mohammed, the prophet of Islam, taught that honey brought a person good luck and health. He was quoted stating: "Honey is a remedy for all diseases."

Consider the following facts about bee products:

- Honeybees visit about two million flowers to make one pound jar of honey.
- A hive of bees flies 55,000 miles to make one jar of honey.
- An average worker bee makes 1/12 of a tablespoon of honey in her life.
- All worker bees are female.
- Bees communicate to one another by dancing, which they can understand even in complete darkness.
- A queen bee can lay up to 3,000 eggs in one day—at a rate of 5 or 6 a minute. That is equal to 175–200 eggs thousand annually.
- One hive may hold up to 80,000 bees—one queen, a few hundred drones (males), and the rest female workers.
- When Alexander the Great died, he was carried back to Greece in a golden coffin filled with honey.
- One gallon of honey equals the combined bee flight distance of going to the moon and back.
- Bees fly an average of 13 to 15 mph.
- Bees from the same hive visit about 225,000 flowers per day. One single bee typically visits between 50 and 1,000 flowers a day, but can visit up to several thousand.
- The average hive temperature is 93.5 degrees Fahrenheit.

- Beeswax production in most hives is about $1^1/2$ to 2 percent of the total honey yield.
- Bees eat about eight pounds of honey to produce one pound of beeswax.
- Honeybees are the only insects that produce food for humans.
- A bee's life span ranges from 3–6 weeks.
- The brain of a worker honeybee is about a cubic millimeter but has the densest neurological tissue of any animal.
- Honeybees are almost the only bees with hairy compound eyes.
- A bee travels an average of 1,600 round trips in order to produce one ounce of honey; up to 6 miles per trip. To produce 2 pounds of honey, bees travel a distance equal to 4 times around the earth.
- Bees have a magnetic band around their brains to help them navigate.
- Bees gather from only one kind of flower at a time. When two different flowers of the same dark purple color grew side by side, bees were noted to nearly collide in air, but never did a bee touch the pollen of the wrong flower.
- Bees are the chief engineers of cross-pollination.
- The honeybee can pollinate at the rate of 30 flowers per minute.
- It takes one bee working eight hours a day for a month to gather 1 teaspoon of bee pollen pellets, which contain over 2.5 billion grains of flower pollen loaded with micronutrients, trace elements, minerals, and antioxidants.
- According to the planetary geological sequence and dating theory, bees are estimated to have survived on Earth for over 150 million years. There are now over 30,000 different bee species.
- Bees produce the only food that will never spoil. Edible honey has been found in Egyptian tombs.

Benefits

Honey, Pollen, Propolis, and Royal Jelly

Bee products are considered to be one of the most spiritual and magical foods on the planet, as well as one of the top superfoods and sources for concentrated nutrition. Consuming high-quality bee products on a

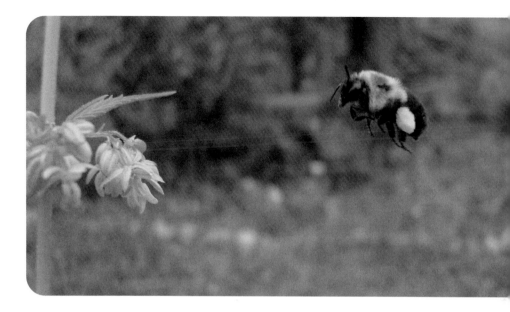

regular basis is highly recommended. Bee products (especially from wild plant and wild tree flowers) are an amazing class of superfood that can complement our health for the rest of our lives.

Honey, in its organic/wild, raw, unfiltered state is rich in minerals, antioxidants, probiotics, enzymes, and is one of the highest-vibration foods on the planet. Honey is also an extremely healing food that provides a very digestible and soothing form of sugar (energy) to the body.

Bee pollen is the most complete superfood found in nature. Containing vitamin B-9 and all twenty-two essential amino acids, it is a delicious-tasting, energy-rich source of complete protein.

Propolis is the substance that seals the hive. It is the protector of the hive. Propolis literally means "for the city." Propolis is a waxy, highly medicinal, immune supporting, and antibacterial substance collected and produced by bees, and has a long history of herbal and alchemical use.

It is important to be aware that the bees from which nonorganic and non-wild honeys and pollens (especially if they are not raw) are collected are often inhumanely treated by corporate honeymakers. This includes feeding the bees high fructose corn syrup (rather than leaving them a portion of their own honey to consume), smoking out the hives, spraying toxic nicotine-based pesticides on the plants/trees from which the bees gather pollen, and a variety of other unsustainable practices.

In light of the recent bee colony collapse disorder and pollination crisis, which, by the way, is primarily affecting the nonorganic bee industry, it is important to support those beekeepers that interact with their bees kindly and lovingly by using organic (nonchemical) methods of beekeeping.

Honey

Made from the nectar that bees sip from flower blossoms, honey is a universal medicine, sweetener, and nutrient resource. The tremendous amount of research conducted on honey in Russia indicates that raw, unprocessed honey is nature's richest source of live healing enzymes and that it increases reflexes, mental alertness, and even IQ! Some types of Lehua and Noni honeys from Hawaii (NoniLand™), Manuka honeys from the New Zealand rainforests, and Sidr honeys from Yemen have been shown to have antifungal, antibiotic, and antiviral effects.

Whenever possible, we recommend that you choose wild honey. We don't have enough wild food in our diet, and wild honey is easy to come by, easy to store, easy to consume, and easy to travel with.

Fresh, wild food has more vitality and more rejuvenating factors. Ten thousand years ago we all ate 100 percent wild food—we just foraged for whatever we could find, we didn't grow anything, there was no agriculture. We know that our teeth and bone mineralization were vastly better in those days. Since the advent of agriculture, our bone mineralization has been gradually decreasing.

All honey should be eaten raw, as cooked honey has no enzymes. Honey can be taken with other mineral-rich superfoods to increase mineral absorption.

Prescription Honey

Honey has been shown to provide relief for, or to cure, a number of different disorders, including, but not limited to: diarrhea, ulcers, infections, irritable bowel syndrome (IBS), gastrointestinal problems, cancer, and staphylococcus (staph) infections.

Infectious diseases caused by bacteria that honey has antibiotic effects upon include the following: anthrax, diphtheria, urinary tract infections, ear infections, meningitis, respiratory infections, sinusitis, pneumonia, tuberculosis, infected animal bites, typhoid, dysentery, abscesses, boils, carbuncles, impetigo, tooth decay, puerperal fever, scarlet fever, sore throat, and cholera.

Honey can also be used topically to heal wounds (especially Manuka honey—the higher the "active number," the more healing and nutritious). A number of different types of wounds have been successfully treated with honey, including abrasions, abscesses, bed sores, burns, burst abdominal wounds following cesarean delivery, cancrum, cervical ulcers, chilblains, cracked nipples, cuts, diabetic foot ulcers and other diabetic ulcers, a fistula, foot ulcers in lepers, infected wounds arising from trauma, large septic wounds, leg ulcers, malignant ulcers, sickle cell ulcers, skin ulcers, surgical wounds, wounds to the abdominal wall and perineum, and varicose ulcers.

The medicinal benefits of honey are due to honey's antibacterial properties and its moisture-retaining properties. Side effects: None.

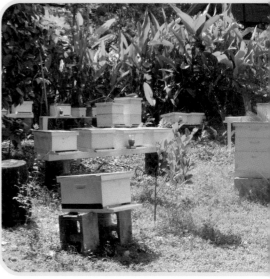

However, honey is inappropriate for children under the age of one due to potential contamination with botulism. And toxic honeys are possible if collected from toxic pollens. Though it is rare, if you are new to keeping bees, please check with your local beekeeping association to see if the potential for toxic pollen exists in your area.

Purines and Blood Sugar

Our cells convert food into energy (ATP) in part by glycolysis. Some people (slow oxidizers) have a slow glycolysis cycle, so they need more carbohydrates due to a lower production of glucose and pyruvate.

The glycolysis cycle of "fast oxidizers" is fast. It is recommended that fast oxidizers reduce foods high on the glycemic index (hybridized foods and food extracts too rich in sugar) and increase high-purine foods, which include high-protein foods such as chlorella and bee pollen.

Blood Sugar Disorders: Cancer, Candida

Special Note: If you have a blood sugar problem or are suffering from a critical health condition, it is a good idea to stay away from honey, agave, sucanat, high fructose corn syrup, evaporated cane juice, any sweeteners, and any kind of sugar for at least two or three months and then reevaluate at that time. It is never a good idea for anyone with a history of cancer to have a lot of sugar in their diet of any type, even from a raw source such as fruit, honey, or agave.

Bee Pollen

Bee pollen is an alkaline food considered by nutritionists to be one of the most complete foods found in nature.

Benefits of bee pollen include:

- High antioxidant levels that help increase longevity by neutralizing free radicals. Antioxidants also help make herbs work more effectively.
- Potent aphrodisiac and fertility-improving properties. Pollen can reduce prostate problems as it rejuvenates sexual organs due to its content of seminal substances. People who suffer from low blood pressure can be subject to deficiencies in sex glands. Pollen increases blood pressure in these types of individuals, especially when taken with kelp, and may increase hormone levels and sexual strength.
- Bee pollen increases strength, endurance, energy, and speed. It provides a quicker recovery from exercise; returns heart rate to normal; and improves endurance for repeat exertion. Bee pollen increases muscle growth and definition. The British Sports Council recorded increases in strength by as high as 40 to 50 percent in those taking bee pollen regularly. Even more astounding, the British Royal Society has reported height increases in adults who take pollen. Antti Lananaki, coach of the Finnish track team that swept the Olympics in 1972, revealed, "Most of our athletes take pollen food supplements. Our studies show it

significantly improves their performance. There have been no negative results since we have been supplying pollen to our athletes."

- Pollen reduces the production of histamine, thus neutralizing many allergies.
- The extraordinary presence of B vitamins in pollen builds up our stress-defense shield, increases longevity, helps clear acne, and assists in reversing aging and wrinkling.
- Helps relieve type 2 diabetes symptoms by restoring mineral and metabolic deficiencies.
- More than forty research studies document the therapeutic efficacy and safety of bee pollen. Clinical tests show that orally ingested bee

Longevity, Bee Pollen, and Russia

Long lives are attained by bee pollen users; it is one of the original treasure-houses of nutrition and medicine. Each grain contains every important substance that is necessary to life.

> —Dr. Naum Petrovich Joirich, chief scientist at the Soviet Academy in Vladivostok (1975)

In 1945 a report from Russian biologist Nicholas Tsitin was published stating that of the one hundred and fifty Russian centenarians who replied to a questionnaire inquiring about their age, occupation, and principal foods, all replied that honey was their main food staple. Further investigation by the Longevity Institute of the USSR revealed that they ate not only honey, but bee pollen and other hive products as well.

Honeybee pollen is the richest source of vitamins found in Nature in a single food. Even if bee pollen had none of its other vital ingredients, its content of rutin alone would justify taking at least a teaspoon daily, if for no other reason than strengthening the capillaries. Pollen is extremely rich in rutin and may have the highest content of any source, plus it provides a high content of the nucleics RNA [ribonucleic acid] and DNA [deoxyribonucleic acid].

> —Institute of Apiculture, Taranov, Russia

pollen particles are rapidly and easily absorbed since they pass directly from the stomach into the blood stream. Within two hours after ingestion, bee pollen is found in the blood, in cerebral spinal fluids, and in urine.

- Pollen has also been noted to assist in helping the following conditions: anemia, constipation, colitis, sinusitis, asthma, and bronchitis.
- Pollen is a source of eighteen vitamins, including nearly all B vitamins (except B12) as well as C, D, and E; rutin (an enzyme catalyst par excellence); carotenes including xanthophyll and beta-carotene; lecithin/choline; all the essential amino acids (twenty-two amino acids in total); fourteen fatty acids including essential fatty acids; eleven carbohydrates ranging from polysaccharides to simple sugars; nucleic acids such as RNA, DNA; steroid hormone substances, a plant hormone similar to the human pituitary called gonadotropin; 15 percent lecithin, and we are still discovering more.
- According to research by doctors from France, Italy, and the USSR, pollen is one of the richest sources of bioavailable protein in nature. Pollen is approximately 25 percent protein. Gram for gram, pollen contains an estimated five to seven times more protein than meat, eggs, or cheese. Because the protein in pollen is in a predigested form, it is easy to assimilate.

Pollen is the reproductive material of the plant world. It is made up of noble substances (trace mineral elements) that have been drawn up, or levitated into, the seminal point of the plant (the flower). Pollen is also abundant in major minerals and trace minerals. It may contain up to sixty elements, including barium, boron, calcium, copper, gold, iodine, iron, magnesium, iron, manganese, phosphorus, potassium, selenium, silicon, sulfur, sodium, and zinc.

In 1981 gold was found in honeybee pollen in amounts as high as 0.9 parts per million (dry weight). Two plants (in British Columbia, Canada) were isolated that could conceivably provide gold in the diet, either to honeybees or perhaps directly: *Phacelia sericea* and *Dryas drummondii*, which carry twenty-five to fifty times as much gold as any other plants with which they are associated.

The overall mineral makeup of pollen is still open to scientific debate.

Most researchers on the subject now agree that a fraction of pollen ranging from 1 to 3 percent of the dried mineral matter consists of unidentified compounds and mineral material. I believe that even the identified fraction of minerals may be misrepresented as carbon when it really consists of something else. That "something else" consists of compounds containing Ormus minerals probably present in polysaccharide carbon chains. These Ormus elements are the mineral elements discovered by David Radius Hudson and now known to occupy a third, newly discovered dimension of Mendeleev's Periodic Table of the Elements. These elements are metals in extremely small atom clusters where the Coulomb force becomes strong enough to overcome forces that cause metal-to-metal atomic covalent bonding. This flips the metal into a substance that appears to the eye to be more like silicon. These Ormus elements possess extraordinary longevity, healing, rejuvenation, neurological, and psychic-enhancing properties.

At least 2 percent of the contents of honeybee pollen has yet to be isolated and identified. The individual pollen grain is encased in two protective coatings. The exine, composed of sporo-pollen and cellulose, is known to be acid-resistant, and has withstood temperatures in excess of 300 degrees C. Beneath this is the thinner, intine layer, which preserves oil and starch.

Pollen contains up to eleven different major enzymes, including diatase, phosphatase, and transferase, as well as high amounts of catalase, amylase, and pectase (a pectin-splitting enzyme), all of which aid in digestion. Just 130 milligrams of bee pollen can help assist in the digestion of three pounds of food, thanks to pollen's enzymatic properties. Experiments show that those who take bee pollen decrease their daily intake of food by 15 to 20 percent.

Royal Jelly

Synthesized from the combination of pollen and honey within the bodies of a special group of young nurse bees, royal jelly is one of the most magical and least understood superfoods in the world. Secreted from the pharyngeal glands, royal jelly is a thick, milky substance that is the only determining factor in the development of a queen bee from an otherwise ordinary larva. Of all of the superfoods, royal jelly is definitely one of the most intriguing, both nutritionally and effectively! Consider the following:

> The greater nutritional significance of Royal Jelly is the fact that the anatomical and functional differentiation of the female larvae is totally dependent upon the nature of their diet in their early development stage. In the larvae stage, they are absolutely identical and feed on Royal Jelly for the first three days after hatching. The fertilized eggs give rise to females which are either sexually immature small worker bees or large, fertile Queens. From the fourth day on, only the special larvae selected to become the Queen continues to be fed with Royal Jelly throughout her entire life, while the worker bees are fed on regular honey and pollen. The fascinating discovery by apiculturalists was that nutrition was the only distinctive difference between the worker bees and the Queen. The Queen Bee is a mother of a quarter of a million bees, and amazingly lays over 2,000 eggs in a single day, a total more than twice her own body weight. The life span of the Queen lasts four to five years, contrary to the considerably shorter life of workers—an average of 3 months or less.
>
> —Excerpted from the article "Fresh Royal Jelly" by Y.S. Royal Jelly and Honey Farm (available on their website, www.yahwehsaliveandwell.com)

Throughout history, many cultures and traditions worldwide have considered royal jelly to be "the fountain of youth and beauty." It is rejuvenating and regenerating for the body, inhibiting the aging process, maintaining skin tone, promoting sexual vitality, alleviating arthritis pain, and acting as an antidepressant, along with many other significant health benefits:

- Royal jelly is known as a rejuvenator, containing B5 and other B vitamins plus amino acids, potassium, magnesium, calcium, zinc, iron, and manganese. It is also a powerful energy supplement; its stimulating effect has been compared to caffeine, without the negative side effects.
- Royal jelly is the second-richest natural source of pantothenic acid (vitamin B5) and contains as much as 50 percent protein, 20 percent carbohydrates, and 14 percent fat.

- Royal jelly is the richest source of acetylcholine, an important fluid in the regulation of nerve impulses between nerve fibers, which enhances our ability to think clearly. Royal jelly is so effective in this area that it is known to help those suffering from Alzheimer's disease.
- Royal jelly is also extremely effective in treating glandular and hormonal imbalances, including those caused by menstrual or prostate problems. In addition to its rejuvenating effect on sight and memory loss, royal jelly aids in the fight against heart disease, including arteriosclerosis and angina.
- A study published in 1960 by the American Association for Cancer Research Inc. found that "whole royal jelly, when pre-mixed with tumor cells before inoculation, has been shown to inhibit completely the development of transplantable AKR leukemia and of three lines of mouse ascitic tumors." This is a significant result!

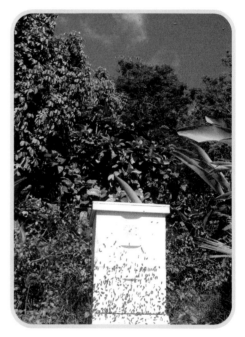

Royal jelly is so complex in its nature that although many investigations have been conducted into its chemical composition and pharmacological properties, scientists have not yet been able to fully analyze nor synthesize it in a laboratory. Royal jelly remains scientific mystery in many regards.

Propolis

The potential for disease to spread inside a hot, crowded hive is high. Millions of years ago, bees solved this problem by gathering the sticky resins, which we know as propolis, from tree buds and bark. Trees exude this resin in order to heal and repair damage and prevent disease. The bioflavonoids in propolis have powerful antibiotic, antifungal, and antibacterial effects.

Bees use it to varnish the cells of the honeycomb, as a glue to seal up cracks, and to create doorways. Propolis protects the bees against bacteria and viruses, and is collected by humans for use as an antibacterial, antifungal, and antibiotic. Unlike penicillin, propolis is all natural and will not produce bad reactions. In biblical times propolis was known as myrrh and was highly prized for its medicinal properties.

> Propolis has long been used as a natural remedy and it is thought that it's the numerous flavonoids which it contains that account for its wound healing benefits. Some studies suggest that it may be used against bacteria and viruses and other microorganisms when applied to infected areas topically. Propolis has antimicrobial action on both gram-positive and gram-negative microorganisms. It contains constituents that increase membrane permeability and inhibit bacterial motility. It is commonly used for wound infection and other illnesses.
>
> —Excerpt from NaturalNews.com's article, "Bee Propolis: Nature's Healing Balm With Immune Boosting Properties" by Katherine East

Propolis is a rich source of minerals, amino acids, fats, vitamins C and E, provitamin A, and B-complex. Propolis is also extraordinarily rich in bioflavonoids and amino acids. The bioflavonoids mend and strengthen the blood vessels and capillaries. In the congested beehive, propolis and royal jelly employ their antibiotic, antimicrobial, anti-inflammatory and antibacterial properties to inhibit undesirable bacteria and promote helpful bacteria. These are all properties that have all been supported by scientific research.

Hundreds of chemical properties have been identified in propolis, which differs from hive to hive, depending upon the environment in which the bees live and the time of day the propolis was collected. All these factors make propolis exceedingly complex, which is why no one has attempted to synthesize the product. It is natural and cannot be patented, and therefore research into the substance is limited regarding its clinical benefits. Consider the following:

> A study was done on the effects of bee propolis on Recurrent Aphthous Stomatitis (RAS)—also known as canker sores—at the Harvard School

of Dental Medicine. Canker sores are an ulcerative disorder of the oral cavity. They have no cure and medicine used to prevent further outbreaks and relieve pain comes with its own set of dangerous side effects. Bee propolis was evaluated as a potential remedy to reduce the number of mouth ulcer outbreaks. There were two groups of patients, one group who took a placebo capsule and the other group who took a propolis capsule. Patients who took the propolis capsule showed a significant decrease in the number of outbreaks of mouth ulcers. Another great effect of the propolis was that the patients reported a definite improvement in their quality of life. This would likely be due to the immune boosting effects that propolis has with its high levels of B-vitamin complex and notable quantities of vitamin C, E, and beta-carotene.

—Excerpt from NaturalNews.com's article "Bee Propolis: Nature's Healing Balm With Immune Boosting Properties" by Katherine East

Propolis has also been used to treat a wide variety of other conditions ranging from arthritis to allergies to asthma. It has even been shown to be effective against MRSA, the antibiotic-resistant bacteria that endangers patients in many hospitals.

What to Look For . . .

Bee Product Types

Honey: the great spiritual, alchemical gift that Mother Nature offers us. Select honeys that are raw, preferably organic, and packaged in glass.

Unique Honey Varieties and Bee Product Types:
NoniLand™ honey: This is the greatest of the dark, amber-colored honeys. This type of honey is found only on the north shores of the Hawaiian Island chain. It is rich in antimicrobial material derived from noni pollen, lehua pollen, and in Ormus minerals in other local north-shore pollens.

Manuka honey: Manuka honeys from New Zealand sometimes are labeled with Active 8+, 10+, 13+, etc. ratings, which are indicators of topical antibiotic power. The higher the rated number, the more powerful the antibiotic effect of the honey when applied to the skin. Look for a high Active + rating if you are using the honey to treat burns or are ingesting the honey to fight back ulcers or an *H. pylori* infection of the stomach.

Honeydew honey: This is another New Zealand honey that is made entirely from tree sap instead of pollen.

Honey with cappings: This honey is capped with bee pollen, royal jelly, propolis, and some beeswax (pieces of the hive). Children tend to love it.

Bee pollen (fresh or dried): Bee pollen is essentially all of the mineral matter inside of flowers that the honeybees gather (they play around inside the flower to collect it) and bring back to the hive on their wings and legs. Pollen grains are microscopic in size and bees collect millions of these individual grains, connecting them with nectar into small pellets. Beekeepers collect the pollen from the bees by placing a mesh collection device at the entrance to the hive that the bees go through. This device gathers between 10 and 50 percent of the pollen that the bees are carrying into a tray below, leaving a sufficient amount for the hive's needs.

When choosing pollen, choose either fresh pollen or look for pollen that has been dried at a hive's natural temperature or less (not above 38° C or 96° F) by the use of dehumidifiers and air coolers in an airtight room. This way the pollen retains its complete nutritional value. Dried pollen needs to be dried to less than 10 percent moisture to stop natural fermentation and spoilage.

Bee pollen, as sold, appears as granular particles that are usually the size of sesame or flaxseeds. Fresh bee pollen is a delightful treat. Fresh bee pollen often has a soft, light, fluffy texture and the taste is full and rich. Dried bee pollen is dehydrated and its grains become harder in texture.

Fresh or dried bee pollen can be preserved in a highly nutritious state if stored in the freezer. The pollen will keep for up to eleven years. This means that bees can still use frozen pollen as food for up to eleven years! The pollen does not actually freeze, possibly due to its low moisture content of 3 percent. Refrigerated pollen does not keep as well because its moisture content can increase, especially if removed regularly from the refrigerator.

The best pollen has a variation of colored granules, ranging across the color spectrum.

Royal jelly: Fresh royal jelly can be frozen or at least refrigerated to preserve its healing and nutritive properties over weeks and months.

Propolis extracts: These product types are usually liquefied in alcohol or extracted in alcohol then put into glycerine. These are usually sold as immune system boosting products.

Propolis eyedrops: This is an excellent eye-cleansing product for individuals looking to use a natural product instead of synthetic eyedrops.

How to Use Bee Products

Honey

Honey is generally not recommended for children under the age of one. Rarely, honey can be contaminated with botulism. This is an organism that can be dangerously toxic to children under the age of one. Even though this is an extremely rare phenomenon, caution is still advised.

Honey can be applied topically to all degrees of burns and abrasions. The labeling of certain New Zealand honeys with Active 3+, Active 10+, Active 18+, etc. ratings is done to denote the topical strength of these honeys.

The aforementioned high Active #+ rated honeys are more effective against *Heliobacter pylori,* a pathogenic microbe organism that has been shown to cause ulcers. Three tablespoons of this type of honey on an empty stomach would be the dosage at least once a day, preferably twice a day, to improve ulcers.

Bee Pollen

Bee pollen can be mixed with honey (and/or royal jelly), consumed by itself as a snack, or blended into smoothies, elixirs, and desserts.

Suggested usage for raw bee pollen

Start by using one tablespoon of bee pollen each day for children over five or adults. Increase serving if desired. Bee pollen blends well with

The Healing Power of Bee Stings

I personally know of many who believe the best and fastest arthritis relief comes from honeybee venom. Some arthritic beekeepers actually annoy bees into stinging the hurting parts of their bodies—ankles, knees, hands and wrists, particularly. Beekeeper Charles Mraz investigated many cases of bee-sting treatment for arthritis and found no recorded instance of allergic reaction to the venom. He believed that most arthritics are not usually allergic to bee venom. From around the world have come thousands of testimonials and reports from doctors, beekeepers, and ordinary people from all walks of life, claiming relief from the symptoms of rheumatic conditions and arthritis by the use of bee sting venom. Why bee venom works this way is not well understood. Some scientists say the bee venom triggers a reaction in the body in which chemicals and perhaps antibodies are released to neutralize the poison and counteract its effects. The assumption is that the body's biological response to the bee venom relieves the symptoms of rheumatic conditions and arthritis, almost as a "side effect"—a desirable side effect. Researchers are trying to find out why bee venom works so they can duplicate its effectiveness in a more controlled and systematic way.

— Bernard Jensen, PhD, *Bee Well Bee Wise with Bee Pollen, Bee Propolis, Royal Jelly*

smoothies or other drinks, or it may be eaten plain as a snack food by the spoonful. For an especially sweet and energizing treat, try dipping a cacao bean in honey, and then sprinkling it with bee pollen and maca!

Warning: On first trying pollen, some people may occasionally experience minor gastrointestinal irritation and a laxative effect due to the richness of the substance. Another potential, yet rare, allergic reaction can involve swelling, heart palpitations, and minor to moderate difficulty in breathing. For those who are new to enjoying pollen, it's wise to start out with a small dosage, about 1/4 teaspoon, and work up from there.

Royal Jelly

Royal jelly is extremely potent. Consuming just half a teaspoon daily is effective to achieve longevity and to receive a solid dosage of B vitamins—especially vitamin B5.

Propolis

Propolis extracts (in alcohol or glycerine) can be added to water by the drop, or droppered directly into the mouth to improve the immune system, especially during a bout of the flu or during a throat infection. Propolis eyedrops are also available and can be used to replace conventional eyedrops. Because propolis products vary in concentration, use each product as directed.

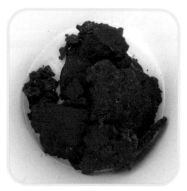

Honey, Bee Pollen, Royal Jelly, and Propolis Recipes

Sweet Superfood Cookie Crumbles

> 1 tbsp. bee pollen
>
> 1 tbsp. açai berry powder
>
> 1/4 tbsp. purple corn extract powder
>
> 1/4 tbsp. mesquite meal
>
> 1/2 tbsp. spirulina
>
> 1 tbsp. coconut cream (not oil)
>
> 1 tsp. raw honey (solidified, white honey works best)

If desired, add 1/2 tsp. cacao powder for chocolate flavor

Mash all ingredients together until a crumbly paste is achieved. Spread on a sheet and dehydrate in a dehydrator or oven until they reach cookie consistency. (The dehydrator should be set at 115 degrees Fahrenheit and let to run until the crumbles are dry. If you have an oven, set it at the

(continued on next page)

lowest temperature and check the crumbles every 10–15 minutes until they are dehydrated.)

Bee-Loving Aphrodisiac Balls

Serves: All Lovers

In a food processor lightly blend:

1/4–1/2 cup dried mulberries

1 cup hempseed

After just a few seconds, just until they are partially soft and grated, place the mixture in a large bowl and add:

8 oz. raw coconut butter (not oil)

1/2 cup shredded dried coconut flakes

3–4 tbsp. maca and/or red maca

1 tsp. cinnamon powder

1/4–1/2 tsp. Celtic sea salt

powder from 12 capsules of cistanche

1/2 cup cacao nibs

1/2 cup tocotrienols

1/2 clove of nutmeg (grate fresh)

3–4 tbsp. bee pollen

1 tbsp. royal jelly

2 tsp. suma powder

1/4 cup lucuma powder

1–2 tsp. ginseng powder (or several squirts in tincture form)

Powder from 6 capsules of cordyceps mushroom

Powder from 6 capsules of ho shou wu

2–3 tbsp. powdered marine phytoplankton

1/4 cup coconut oil

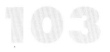

2 tbsp. raw NoniLand™ honey

3 raw vanilla beans (scrape out powder inside, do not use outside skin)

Massage all ingredients together by hand until the consistency of cookie dough. If necessary, add a splash or two of spring water or more coconut oil so everything sticks together.

Roll into golf-ball-sized balls, dip each ball in one of the following toppings and feed to the lucky person of your choice:

Maca powder

Coconut flakes

Cinnamon powder

Cacao nibs

Bee pollen

Shot o' Gold Tonic

1 dropperful of Ormus Gold

1 dropperful propolis tincture

1 oz. Colloidal Gold

2 tsp. fresh pressed ginger juice

1–2 tsp. raw NoniLand™ honey healing honey

1 tsp. bee pollen

1 oz. Orgono Living Silica

1 squirt Dr. Patrick Flanagan's Crystal Energy

1 tbsp. powdered marine phytoplankton

Optional for extra magic: 1 dropperful of goji berry extract tincture or 1 tbsp. goji berry extract powder

Mix all ingredients together in a glass (not a blender), stir, drink it down, and you are gold to go!

Guru Power Goo

2 tbsp. bee pollen

2 tsp. royal jelly

2 tbsp. raw NoniLand™ honey

2–4 droppersful of propolis tincture

Mix all ingredients together in bowl and enjoy!

High-vibe variations: Add in a few spoonfuls of whichever of the following ingredients strike your fancy—let your creative culinary genius go wild!

Cacao nibs (or whole beans)

Wild jungle peanuts

Brazil nuts (chopped)

Hempseed

Shelled pecans

Goji berries

Hunza raisins

Dried mulberries

Dried (chopped) figs

Dried (chopped) dates

Superfood Skinny Dippers

Place each of the following six ingredients in their own bowls, and decadently dip away with the cacao bean!

cacao beans

Manuka or NoniLand™ honey

royal jelly

maca

bee pollen

spirulina

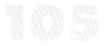

Bee Royal Spread

On top of your favorite flax crackers, or raw/sprouted bread, spread:

    1 tbsp. Manuka or NoniLand™ honey

    1 tsp. royal jelly

And then sprinkle on:

    1 tbsp. hempseed

and a pinch of your favorite spice(s), including, but not limited to: cayenne, cinnamon, ginger, curry, Italian seasoning, etc. (optional)

NoniLand™ Lemonade Cleanser

    16 oz. spring water

    2 tbsp. NoniLand™ honey (or more, to taste)

    juice of 1–2 lemons

    1 pinch of Celtic sea salt

    2 tbsp. NoniLand™ noni powder

Combine all ingredients together in a jar and stir until completely mixed together. Chill in refrigerator (or even freezer if you want a sorbet) for an extra-refreshing treat!

"True," he continued, "the Path of Pollen has its dangers, for before there is birth there is labor—if honey, then also sting. But at its completion, it confers upon those who attain it extraordinary control over physical conditions. These include the ability to transmute matter, to heal all diseases, and to prolong the span of human incarnation. The Path of Pollen is our yoga, our means of union and communion with the incredible hidden universe and this beautiful blue-green jewel that is our Earth."

    —The Bee Shaman Bridge speaking to Simon Buxton
      in *The Shamanic Way of the Bee*

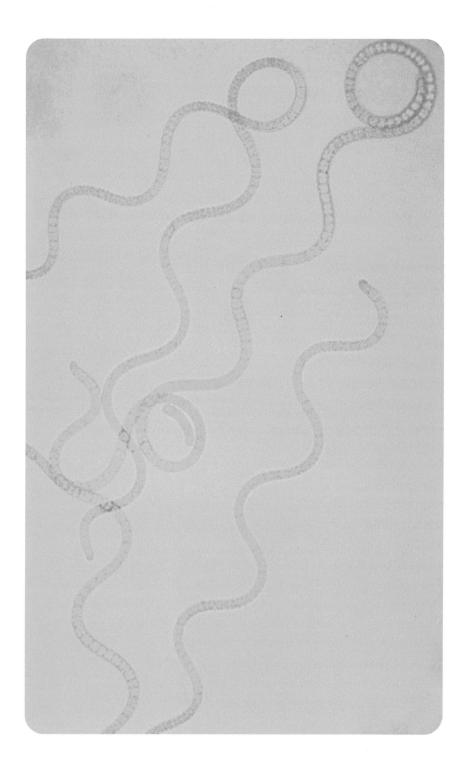

Spirulina
Protein Queen

Latin Names:

Major varieties: *Spirulina pacifica,*
   Spirulina platensis, Spirulina maxima,
   Spirulina fusiformis

Common Names:

Spirulina, *Tecuitlatl* (Aztec), *Dihe* (African)

Superfood Type:

Algae (powder, flakes, or cakes)

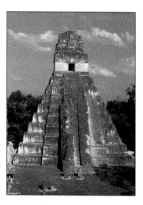

History, Facts, and Legends

Spirulina belongs to an ancient class of single-celled, blue-green spiral algae. At least thirty-five varieties of spirulina still exist in various lakes and waterways across the Earth.

Spirulina are freshwater-growing, alkaline-environment, microscopic algae that have been living on the planet since the appearance of life on Earth. Spirulina form spiraling, helical, microscopic strands that are smaller than the human eye can detect. The name "spirulina" comes from this superfood's spiral character.

Spirulina's green color is derived from chlorophyll and the blue color is derived from the exotic pigment phycocyanin.

As one of the simplest life-forms, spirulina has an extraordinarily long history of helping to sustain and develop the food chain. It is clear that ancient algae and plankton life-forms from the Earth's lakes and oceans

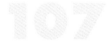

provide the fundamental nutrient and food sources for all life. They are the basis and beginning of the food chain. Through photosynthesis algae and plankton convert sunlight into pure protein, fatty acids, carbohydrates, and nearly every other nutrient essential to life.

Spirulina are hardy survivors. Some spirulina varieties survive in a dormant state even when water evaporates. They can dry out on rocks as hot as 160 degrees Fahrenheit. Because of this heat resistance, spirulina retains its nutrients even when exposed to high temperatures during travel and food processing.

Spirulina algae cells grow naturally in warm, alkaline lakes and waterways where toxic organisms cannot endure, so spirulina harvesting can be achieved with a high degree of sterility without contamination from other organisms.

Historically, two civilizations were known to enjoy spirulina on a large scale: the peoples of Mexico City in Central America and those in the area of Lake Chad in Africa.

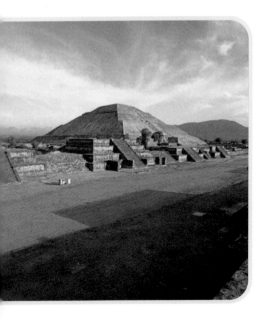

In modern times, significant commercial harvesting of spirulina began in the 1970s, with initial harvests nearing one hundred tons per year. Worldwide production of spirulina is expected to reach 220,000 tons annually by the year 2020.

American Spirulina

Spirulina was the primary protein source for citizens of Mexico City for several thousand years. Spirulina grows wildly in some of the lakes that once surrounded Mexico City, now engulfed by the sprawl of the world's biggest city. One of these, Lake Texcoco, still produces some of the world's best spirulina. The last great Aztec dynasties, before the arrival of the Spanish in 1519, revered spirulina as a superfood and were known to mix it with chocolate. Chocolate (cacao) and spirulina have been eaten together since Mexico City was founded. The Aztecs knew spirulina by their word *tecuitlatl*.

The spirulina currently grown on the southern tip of the Big Island of Hawaii is a variety that was isolated from the streams and waterways of Hawaii. This is *Spirulina pacifica* and it is grown by the spirulina farming company Cyanotech. While there is no record of the ancient Hawaiians consuming this spirulina that I know of, consuming spirulina with Polynesian foods such as coconuts, noni, and turmeric indicates the obvious synergy between these tropical foods and spirulina.

African Spirulina

African peoples living near Lake Chad have been consuming spirulina since the beginning of human inhabitation in the area. They call their wild spirulina *dihe.* The spirulina is sifted off the top of the lake, dried on rocks or racks, and sold in the regional markets.

Benefits

Spirulina contains an astounding array of nutrients, including chlorophyll, protein, vitamins, major minerals, trace minerals, essential fatty acids, nucleic acids (RNA and DNA), polysaccharides, and a vast spectrum of antioxidants. Spirulina is so rich in nutrition that it is believed by some that you could live on spirulina alone for quite some time.

Spirulina:
- Is an algae superfood that consists of 65–71 percent protein (the highest concentration of protein found in any food)
- Is a complete protein source. It contains all eight essential amino acids, and eighteen amino acids in total
- Is rich in vitamins A (beta-carotene), B1, B2, B6, E, and K
- Is an abundant natural source of chlorophyll, salts, phytonutrients, and enzymes
- Provided the primary protein requirements for millions of people in Mexico City for an estimated five thousand years!

- Is the best source of gamma-linolenic acid (GLA), an anti-inflammatory essential fatty acid necessary for a healthy nervous system
- Contains phycocyanin, a potent health-building pigment that also gives spirulina its unique blue tint

Protein

Spirulina contains the highest concentration of protein (by weight) of any food known, between 65 and 71 percent protein, depending upon the variety.

Protein is not just useful for building muscle and strength; it is also useful for endurance, balanced blood sugar, balanced brain chemistry, neurological health, rapid healing, building strong bones, and nearly every other aspect of healthy living.

The challenge we face in deriving our protein from animals is that "high-protein" animal foods involve killing, gruesome slaughterhouses, environmentally destructive factory farming, chemicals, pesticides, hormones, antibiotics, Orwellian breeding and genetic modification programs, government subsidization, and more. All of these animal foods must then be cooked to death in order to kill pathogenic *E. coli* and *Salmonella* organisms that often contaminate such products.

In his book *Rainbow Green Live-Food Cuisine*, Dr. Gabriel Cousens cites research done by the Max Planck Institute on protein. This research demonstrates that 50 percent of the protein present in food is lost when our food is cooked. Given this, all listed protein values for meat (other than sushi) are probably inflated by a factor of two.

Spirulina, unlike animal foods, is a pure, raw source of complete protein. It is never cooked and never needs to be cooked. The spirulina organism converts sunlight to protein more efficiently than any other living thing. Switching from animal protein to spirulina protein is one of the most effective ways to conserve natural resources and improve the environment. Spirulina protein is also more readily absorbed than animal protein because it can be easily blended into water, beverages, smoothies, and shakes without coagulation or heat. Each gram of spirulina protein is four times more absorbable than the same gram of protein in beef.

Spirulina

Spirulina yields two hundred times more protein per acre than beef. Spirulina does not deplete any topsoil and can actually improve topsoil if used as a fertilizer ("vegan manure"). One kilo (2.2 pounds) of beef protein causes 145 kilos (320 pounds) of topsoil loss.

As for water savings, spirulina uses only 2 percent of the water required for beef protein. Spirulina uses about six gallons (23 liters) of water for a 0.35 ounce (10 gram) serving. Cow's milk uses 65 gallons (246 liters), a chicken's egg uses 136 gallons (36 liters), and beef uses a shocking 1,303 gallons of water for a 0.35 ounce (10 gram) serving.

Balanced Brain Chemistry

Full-spectrum protein sources such as spirulina are known for their importance in balancing brain chemistry. The absence of certain protein building blocks known as amino acids may create a cascade of problems. For example, the absence of the amino acid tryptophan in the diet will lead to a deficiency in serotonin (which the body creates from tryptophan). Serotonin is essential for generating feelings of well-being. Serotonin is also a "stress-defense shield" that helps us cope with hardships. A serotonin deficiency has been associated with depression, chronic stomach problems, and neurological disorders. We can readily see from just this example the importance of just one amino acid.

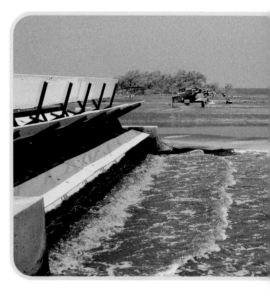

Purity

As exposure levels of artificial chemicals, pesticides, and radioactive materials continue to increase, more and more people are becoming interested in eating lower on the food chain (rather than eating animal products such as meat and dairy that are high on the food chain where toxins accumulate). This means eating more and more plants, especially algae.

The effects of eating animal products—excessive cholesterol, saturated fat, weight gain, and ingestion of artificial chemicals (pesticides, injected hormones, animal vaccinations, etc.) if you're not eating organic—are causing millions of people to seek refuge in more humane, sustainable, and pure vegetarian, vegan, and raw-food approaches to diet and lifestyle. Of course, vegetarian sources of protein must be found, and spirulina is at the top of the list.

Blood Builder

Experience has taught me that the studies and anecdotal stories about spirulina helping alleviate anemia, increasing hemoglobin, improving blood quality, and increasing red blood cell formation are true. Why?

- Spirulina contains as much iron as red meat.
- Spirulina contains high concentrations of chlorophyll, a known blood-builder.
- Spirulina is rich in a brilliant blue polypeptide known as phycocyanin. This blue pigment helps induce the production of more stem cells found in bone marrow. Stem cells are the beginning rudimentary cells that can develop into both red and white blood cells. Some Chinese scientists document phycocyanin as stimulating the creation of blood, a process known as *hematopoiesis.*

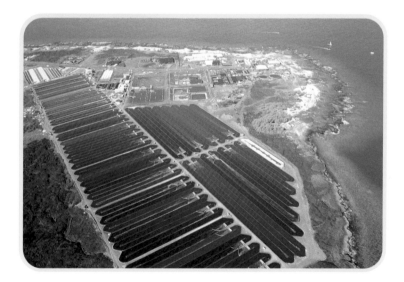

Antioxidants

The antioxidants in spirulina had to protect this algae and its DNA from ultraviolet radiation early in the Earth's history, when the atmosphere was much thinner than it is today and the plants were mostly blue instead of green, due to differences in our sun's spectrum of radiation in the Cambrian geological period. When we ingest spirulina, its antioxidant green-and-blue pigments become available to our cells and thus we become more significantly protected from ultraviolet radiation at the cellular level.

Over the course of time, our DNA is damaged by free radicals generated as a byproduct of normal metabolism and by exposure to toxins and radiation. Damage to our DNA opens the door to illness and accelerates aging. Although our bodies are equipped to continually repair themselves, they can become overwhelmed by too many free radicals, especially as we age. This results in the premature death of healthy cells, which may contribute to a variety of degenerative diseases and the accelerated development of mutated cells that can lead to cancer—unless antioxidants counter the onslaught.

Spirulina contains the following antioxidants:

- Beta-carotene (and other carotenoids). Carotenoids are natural fat-soluble antioxidants that are known to increase life span and improve the immune system.
- Chlorophyll: a blood builder and purifier *par excellence.*
- Zeaxanthin: the most important antioxidant for improving vision.
- Superoxide dismutase (SOD): generally regarded as one of the most important health-enhancing metabolic enzymes and antioxidants.
- Phycocyanin: an extraordinary blue pigment known to help stimulate the production of stem cells. (Note: Color pigments in plants are antioxidants.)

Topical antioxidants protect our skin from excessive sun exposure. For those with sensitive skin, one can create a sunscreen at home by adding spirulina (as needed) to a simple 50/50 mixture of raw organic coconut oil and raw organic cacao butter. The more spirulina added, the greater will be the protection, however, the mixture will continue to become more blue-green, creating a blue-green lotion that may or may not be considered "sexy" at the beach.

Immune System Booster

Spirulina is a powerful tonic for the immune system. In scientific studies of humans, mice, rats, hamsters, chickens, turkeys, cats, and fish, the introduction of spirulina into the diet consistently improves immune system function. Spirulina accelerates production of the humeral aspect of the immune system by helping to increase the production of antibodies and cytokines, including interferons and interleukins, allowing the body to better protect against invasive microbes and viruses.

Spirulina accelerates the production of the cellular immune system by helping to increase the production of bone marrow stem cells, T-fighter cells, macrophages, B-cells, and the anti-cancer natural killer (NK) cells. Scientists have almost universally observed that spirulina causes macrophages to increase in population and to become more effective at killing microbes even in spite of stresses from environmental toxins and infectious agents.

Once the production of new immune system cells circulate in the blood, they begin to concentrate in the adenoids (tonsils), appendix, bone marrow, liver, lymph nodes, spleen, and thymus, increasing overall health and immunity.

The primary active phytonutrients in spirulina responsible for improving the immune system include:

- Research indicates that the more beta-carotene you have in your diet, the longer you will live. Plant- and algae-derived beta-carotene inhibits the replication of certain cancers in animals and in humans.
- A type of lipo-polysaccharide known as LPS a long, complex sugar molecule attached to a molecule of fat/oil via a covalent bond.
- The stem-cell-producing blue antioxidant known as phycocyanin.

A double-blind peer-reviewed human study conducted in India and published in *Nutrition and Cancer,* found that the consumption of one gram of spirulina daily for one year resulted in a 45 percent remission of oral precancerous lesions in tobacco chewers compared to a 7 percent response in the placebo group.

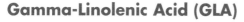
Gamma-Linolenic Acid (GLA)

The richest whole-food sources of GLA are mother's milk, spirulina microalgae, and the seeds of borage, black currant, and evening primrose. GLA is important for growth and development, and is found most abundantly in mother's milk; spirulina is the next-highest whole-food source. We often recommend spirulina for people who were never breast-fed, in order to foster the hormonal and mental development that may never have occurred because of lack of proper nutrition in infancy. The dosage is the amount of oil that provides 150–350 mg GLA daily. A standard 10-gram dosage of spirulina provides 131 mg of GLA.

—Paul Pitchford, *Healing with Whole Foods*

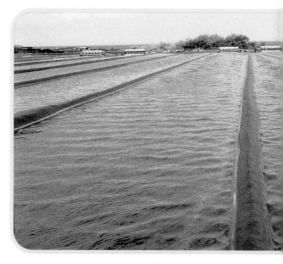

Spirulina is the only green food rich in the essential fatty acid gamma-linolenic acid (GLA). The only other major superfood with concentrations of GLA similar to spirulina is hempseed.

Because it is an essential fatty acid, GLA makes one's skin and hair shiny and strong, yet soft.

GLA has been shown to inhibit the formation of inflammatory prostaglandins and arachidonate metabolites. Spirulina is an excellent superfood to help fight the inflammatory symptoms of arthritis.

GLA may be a contributing factor in spirulina's observed ability to reduce allergies.

Studies showed that 270 children living in highly radioactive areas near Chernobyl had chronic radiation sickness and elevated levels of Immunoglobulin E (IgE), a marker for high allergy sensitivity. Thirty-five preschool children were prescribed 20 spirulina tablets per day (about 5 grams) for 45 days. Consuming spirulina lowered the levels of 2IgE in the blood, which then normalized allergic sensitivities in the body.

In studies with rats, spirulina inhibited allergic reactions by inhibiting the release of histamine in a dose-dependent fashion, again suggesting that GLA may be a primary contributing factor to spirulina's allergy-fighting properties.

Sulfur

Spirulina also contains several bioavailable forms of the mineral sulfur. Sulfur may be detected in spirulina as a "hard-boiled egg" type of taste. A good source of dietary sulfur such as spirulina will improve the immune system, physical strength, flexibility, agility, complexion, hair's luster, speed of healing, and the functionality of your liver and pancreas. Sulfur can also help to rid our tissues of toxins.

The forms of sulfur in spirulina include sulfur-bearing amino acids, sulfoglycolipids, and calcium-spirulan.

Sulfur-bearing amino acids such as cysteine and methionine help the liver and nervous system detoxify poisons. Researchers generally consider spirulina to possess valuable detoxification properties.

Spirulina may help ADHD by removing aluminum, carbon tetrachloride, and other toxins from the body.

—Donald R. Yance, *Herbal Medicine, Healing & Cancer*

Calcium-spirulan is a polymerized sugar molecule unique to spirulina, containing both sulfur and calcium. Hamsters treated with a calcium-spirulan extract had better recovery rates when infected with an otherwise lethal herpes virus. When attacking a cell, a herpes virus first attaches itself to the cell membrane; however, at that point the calcium-spirulan blocks the herpes virus from entering the cell. The virus gets stuck on the membrane and is unable to replicate. It is eventually cleaned off by the immune system.

Vitamin B12

The vitamin B12 in spirulina has not been observed to increase B12 in human blood in clinical research done by Dr. Gabriel Cousens. Therefore, the conclusion, at this point in the research is that even though spirulina contains vitamin B12, it does not increase vitamin B12 in the human body and does not reverse a vitamin B12 deficiency, although it may reverse many symptoms often related to a vitamin B12 deficiency such as anemia.

What to Look For . . .

Spirulina Product Types

Spirulina is usually available as a deep-green, slightly blue, richly pigmented, dry algae powder. Spirulina tastes somewhat like a cross between chlorophyll and fish, with a slightly sulfur-rich aftertaste. When purchasing dried spirulina, look for the following characteristics:

1. Certified organic spirulina is usually, but not always, superior to other types of spirulina. If you have found a nonorganic brand of spirulina that you enjoy, and you are satisfied with the way the spirulina is produced, then stick with it.

2. Select spirulina with a "fresh" smell. When spirulina starts to go bad, it smells sour and rancid.

3. Avoid spirulina brands that use "tableting agents," which help keep spirulina tablets from crumbling to powder. Spirulina naturally clings to itself and can be pressed into tablets without tableting agents.

Below is a list of spirulina product types to look for on the Internet or in your health food store or supplement shop.

Spirulina powder (dried)

Spirulina powder (with lecithin)

Spirulina protein powder products

Spirulina blue pigment extracts

Raw spirulina chocolate bars and spirulina energy bars

How to Use Spirulina

Spirulina is "cooling" and "wet" by nature. This means that if you have a hot, dry metabolism, spirulina is a great food choice for you because spirulina will tend to balance out the tendency to be too hot or dehydrated.

Spirulina's cooling and wet signature also make it a great food for hot, dry climates. This is one of the reasons why Native Americans who lived in pre-Columbian Mexico City used spirulina as their primary source of protein. It is a perfect food for the climate there.

Spirulina can easily be added into superfood smoothies, fresh juices, raw chocolate (cacao) concoctions, homemade salad dressings, and even sprinkled on top of salads. After experimenting with spirulina for a few weeks, you will notice how extraordinary this super-protein is in nutrition, compared to animal protein and/or simple fruits and vegetables.

Recommended Dosages
- Beginner or Child (ages 2–9): 3–5 grams a day
- Normal or Child (ages 10–18): 6–10 grams a day
- Therapeutic dose: 11–20 grams a day
- Super-Athlete dose: as much as 30+ grams a day

Can you have too much spirulina? Like any other food or superfood, this is of course possible. If you have too much, it will simply pass through you. The caloric value of spirulina is so low that it can never be fattening. Spirulina contains approximately four calories per gram.

Spirulina comes in handy for more than just personal nutrition. Recently Sacred Chocolate ordered 404 kilograms of spirulina for our Hawaiian chocolate farm from Cyanotech Corporation, a spirulina growing facility on the Big Island of Hawaii. The company sells "throw away" spirulina that fell on the packaging facility floor, or for some other reason cannot be sold for consumption. We use it as fertilizer instead of manure.

Spirulina Recipes

Spiry Salad Dressing

   1/2 cup organic hempseed

   1 handful fresh dill (stems and everything)

   2–3 cloves garlic (depends how spicy it is)

   2 tbsp. spirulina

   1 tsp. Celtic sea salt

   1 cup fresh spring water

Blend in a high-speed blender until creamy and smooth. Serve on a fresh, garden-picked salad for optimal pleasure!

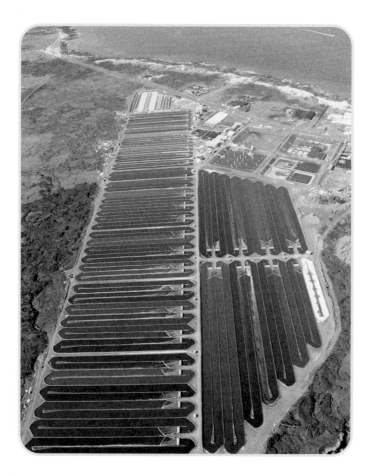

Spirulina-and-Chocolate Balls

1/4 hempseed (ground or whole)

1/2 cup cacao powder

2 tbsp. spirulina

1 tbsp. tocotrienols (optional and delicious)

2 tbsp. coconut oil

3 tbsp. organic or wild, raw honey (already softened is easier)

1 pinch of Celtic sea salt (finely ground)

1 inside of vanilla bean, or 1 tsp. vanilla bean powder

Thoroughly mix with love, roll into little balls, freeze for about 15 minutes, and enjoy.

Delicious tip: drink hemp milk with these amazing spirulina cookie balls.

Amazing Guacamole—Real Mexican Style

2–3 ripe, organic avocados, diced or mashed

1 organic tomato, diced

1 small organic red onion, finely diced

1 handful fresh organic cilantro, finely diced

1 tbsp. spirulina

1 pinch Celtic sea salt

juice of 1 organic lime

Stir gently, preferably with a wooden salad fork, and enjoy!

And of course, the infamous . . .

Mixture of Hempseed, Spirulina, and Celtic Sea Salt

Start off with these amounts, and play around till you find your favorite combination.

  1 cup organic hempseed

  2 tbsp. spirulina

  1 tsp. Celtic sea salt (coarse or fine)

Shake all ingredients in a jar. Snack on this mixture like a trail mix. Use a spoon to dip in.

*All spirulina recipes concocted by Camille "Super Goji Girl" Perrin—tried, tested, and enjoyed by fellow Superheroes.

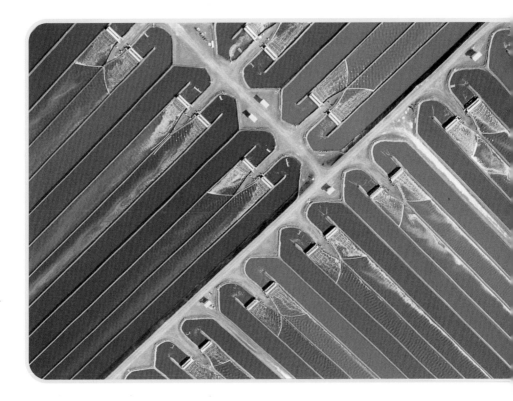

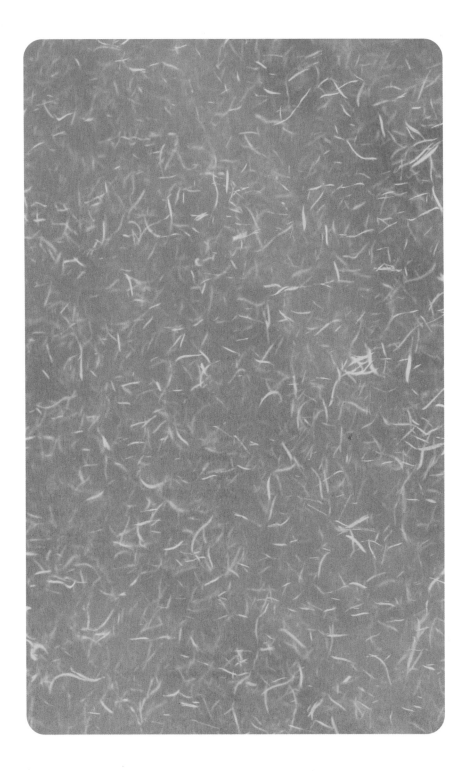

AFA Super Blue-Green Algae

Primordial Food from Klamath Lake, Oregon

Latin Names:

Aphanizomenon flos-aquae

Common Names:

Klamath Lake Blue-Green Algae,
    AFA Blue-Green Algae, Algae,
    Blue-Green Algae, AFA

Superfood Type:

Algae

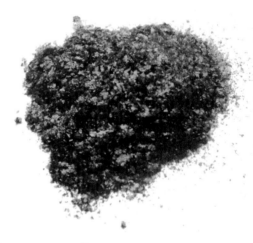

History, Facts, and Legends

Klamath Lake blue-green algae is a form of microalgae phytoplankton that differs from spirulina in that it prefers fresh water as opposed to brackish, salty water. At least forty thousand species of microalgae phytoplankton have been identified, not only including blue-green algae, but also ocean-dwelling marine phytoplankton species, seaweeds, freshwater pond algae, and mosses of many colors.

Microalgae phytoplankton form the basis of the food chain. Fossil evidence indicates they were very likely the first organisms to populate the

Earth and are still here eons later. Some scientists believe microalgae have been on Earth for approximately 2.8 billion years.

Microalgae are responsible for an estimated 80 to 90 percent of the planet's overall food supply and oxygen supply. Microalgae obtain their energy through the process of photosynthesis. It is through algal photosynthesis that the Earth's early atmosphere was converted into its present oxygen-rich state. It seems clear that algae have been the primary developers of the Earth's atmosphere since life appeared on Earth.

Blue-green algae (of the *Cyanophyta* family) are extremely hardy survivors and can adapt to a wide range of light, heat, carbon dioxide levels, oxygen levels, and unique aqueous physical environments. Blue-green algae are the richest sources of chlorophyll found in nature. They photosynthesize better than any plant on Earth.

Blue-green algae are similar in structure to a soft bacteria with chlorophyll, phycocyanin, and other pigments. Like bacteria, blue-green algae are prokaryotes because they lack a membrane-bound nucleus. The genetic information in blue-green algae (DNA and RNA) is easily absorbed by our intestinal flora (friendly bacteria that live in our digestive system). This helps our intestinal bacteria and consequently our bodies digest and connect with the eons-old information contained within blue-green algae, allowing us to improve our immune system and to better adapt to changing conditions in our environment.

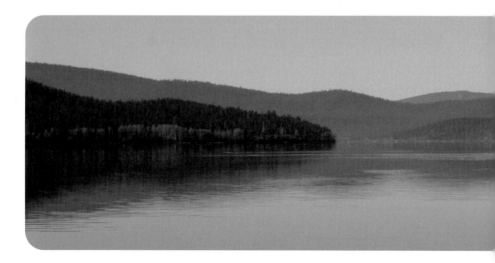

Aphanizomenon flos-aquae (AFA) blue-green algae is a particular type of wild blue-green algae that populates its natural habitat—a giant shallow body of water known as Klamath Lake in Oregon. At 125 square miles, Klamath Lake is the largest lake in Oregon. It is also at a relatively high altitude, 4,139 feet above sea level.

In his booklet *Primordial Food,* Christian Drapeau writes:

> Klamath Lake is located in a relatively undeveloped area, surrounded by publicly owned land such as the Crater Lake National Park, the Winema National Forest, the Lower Klamath National Wildlife Refuge, and the Tule Lake National Wildlife Bird Refuge. With the Cascade Mountains to the west, thousands of square miles of National Park to the north and east, and the city of Klamath Falls located downstream at the southern end of the lake, Klamath Lake is virtually untouched by industrial activity and pollution.

AFA is a nitrogen-fixing algae that draws nitrogen from the atmosphere to build world-class protein. AFA has been harvested, filtered, cleaned, and dried from Klamath Lake for worldwide consumption since the 1970s.

AFA blue-green algae from Klamath Lake has become a popular super-food among health enthusiasts all over the world. Blue-green algae is a wild food with a fantastic array of brain-specific phytochemicals, a huge selection of antioxidants, minerals (especially iron, zinc, selenium, and

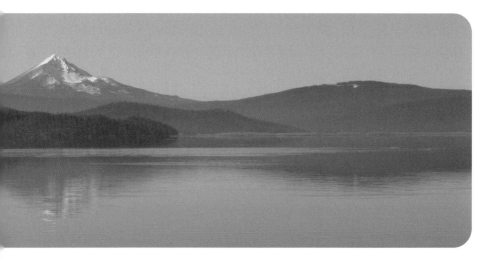

magnesium), amino acids (it is a complete protein), vitamins, enzymes, and many unique nutrients. Blue-green algae is one of the richest food sources of antioxidant compounds, including carotenoids (beta-carotene, lycopene, and lutein), chlorophyll, and phycocyanin.

AFA Blue-Green Algae and Spirulina Compared

- AFA is a wild food harvested from a wild environment. Spirulina is a wild species grown in a controlled environment. Generally this indicates that AFA will contain more minerals than spirulina. Analytical research supports this conclusion.
- AFA contains more chlorophyll. Ten grams of AFA algae contains approximately 300 mg of chlorophyll. A 10-gram portion of spirulina contains approximately 120 mg.
- AFA contains more phycocyanin. AFA blue-green algae has more than twice the phycocyanin (blue pigments) of spirulina: 15 percent versus 7 percent.
- AFA contains more vitamin C. AFA blue-green algae contains more than five times the vitamin C content of spirulina.
- AFA contains more essential fatty acids. AFA blue-green algae is a cold-water algae that insulates itself with essential fatty acids. In warmer, tropical, saltwater pools (where spirulina grows) less of the insulating, essential fatty acids are required.

An initial review of this comparison indicates that AFA blue-green algae is superior to spirulina. However, years of experience have demonstrated to me that spirulina is more friendly to human metabolism and digestion than AFA blue-green algae. Try them both and see what works for you!

Benefits

Aphanizomenon flos-aquae (AFA) blue-green algae are made primarily of soft proteins and polysaccharides that are easily digested by our intestinal bacteria that in turn then feed our blood and cells. This "softness" makes AFA one of the most digestible and utilizable protein foods in all of nature. This "soft" characteristic is unusual for plant cells, but is common for animal cells; this is a reason why blue-green algae are often considered 25 percent animal.

AFA is loaded with chlorophyll (1–2 percent of its dry weight). Chlorophyll helps build our blood due to the presence of the pyrol ring in chlorophyll, which is identical to the pyrol ring found in hemoglobin. Chlorophyll helps fight leukemia as well as certain forms of skin and liver cancer. Additionally, chlorophyll helps to deodorize the bowels.

AFA contains an extraordinarily high concentration of the blue-pigment phycocyanin (15 percent) which helps preload the immune system by stimulating the production of more stem cells from the bone marrow. Stem cells are the basic form of all cells and can be transformed into any cell (including T-cells, NK cells, macrophages, and other immune system cell artillery).

AFA is known to contain an exceptional forty major and trace minerals, picked up from the constant stirring of nearly thirty feet of mineral sediment at the bottom of Klamath Lake. Minerals are the atomic matrix of our bodies and are necessary to build every tissue including our bones, teeth, skin, hair, nails,

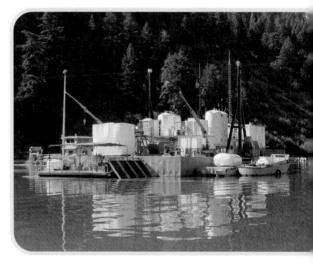

internal organs, muscular system, immune system, and nervous system.

Generally, the more domesticated our food is, the more mineral deficient it becomes. Weston Price's work in *Nutrition and Physical Degeneration* demonstrated that the more one adopts a "civilized" diet, the more quickly mineral deficiency symptoms appear. Mineral deficiencies have been associated with every degenerative and chronic condition known to humankind. The key solution to mineral deficiencies appears to be including wild foods in our diet. AFA is a wild food.

AFA is an excellent source of B vitamins including appreciable amounts of vitamins B1, B2, B3, B5, B6, B9, and B12. In general, B vitamins fight stress by helping to more efficiently convert polysaccharides and other carbohydrates into glucose for immediately available energy, endurance, and stamina.

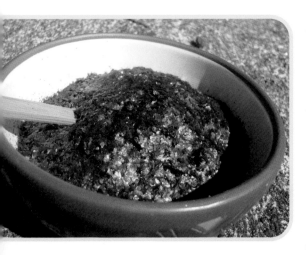

The vitamin B12 found in AFA may or may not be usable by the human body. Dr. Gabriel Cousens's clinical research indicates that the vitamin B12 in AFA does not increase serum B12 levels in human blood, indicating that the B12 in AFA is unavailable. AFA is also an important source of vitamin C.

AFA contains omega-3 fatty acids, including the long-chain omega-3 fatty acid known as docosahexanoic acid (DHA). AFA also contains the phospholipid choline. This makes AFA a brain and nervous system supporting food.

Protein

AFA algae is a complete protein source containing approximately 60 percent protein. Eighteen amino acids (protein building blocks) are present in AFA algae. The protein and amino acids in AFA is in highly assimilable glycoprotein and amino acid peptide forms instead of the lipoprotein form found in animal products such as beef and chicken (which are usually cooked into even more difficult-to-digest forms of protein). Therefore, it takes less energy to digest and utilize algae protein. Additionally, neurotransmitters for brain health can be produced from AFA protein more easily and swiftly due to its ease of digestibility.

Protein is used to construct, maintain, and repair every tissue in our bodies from our bones, teeth, muscles, nerves, glands, heart, blood, liver, skin, hair, and everything in between. A lack of protein is mostly associated with muscular weakness, slow healing, and brain chemistry imbalances. An excess of animal protein is associated with heart disease, kidney disease, cancer, and colon cancer. It is becoming more and more clear that plant-based, complete protein sources are of critical importance for the future—this is exactly what superfoods provide and this is exactly what AFA algae provides.

Some of the free amino acid peptides found in AFA may be responsible for helping to detoxify our bodies of heavy metals. Dr. Gillian McKeith reports in her booklet *Miracle Superfood: Wild Blue-Green Algae* that in her clinical experience AFA algae has been effective in chelating (removing) dangerous, toxic heavy metals such as cadmium, lead, and mercury. She recommends consuming 0.21 to 0.35 ounces (6 to 10 grams) of AFA blue-green algae daily for severe cases of heavy-metal toxicity.

Phycocyanin

The antioxidant phycocyanin is a pigment that provides the intense blue color in blue-green algae. Phycocyanin can constitute up to 15 percent of the dry weight of a blue-green algae harvest; this is approximately twice the concentration of the phycocyanin found in spirulina. The rare, blue-colored phycocyanin helps inhibit the growth of certain cancer colonies, reduces inflammation of the colitis, fights chronic inflammation, supports the liver, protects against free-radical damage, improves the production of neurotransmitters, and aids production of rejuvenating stem cells.

- Phycocyanin operates with our own internal pigment bilirubin to keep the liver functioning at optimal levels.
- Phycocyanin helps with the formation of neurotransmitters by acting to assist in the attachment of one amino acid to another.
- Phycocyanin has been shown to inhibit the enzymes cyclooxygenase (COX-2) and lipoxygenase. COX-2 and lipoxygenase are enzymes associated with the production of inflammatory compounds. When COX-2 and lipoxygenase are inhibited naturally with phycocyanin, the inflammatory and pain-forming reactions in the body are slowed and/or stopped.

Phenylethylamine (PEA)

Also found within AFA algae is a concentrated level of phenylethylamine (PEA), an adrenal and brain chemical naturally synthesized in our bodies from two amino acids: phenylalanine and tyrosine. PEA increases the activity of neurotransmitters (brain chemicals) in parts of the brain that control our ability to pay attention and stay alert. Elevated PEA levels occur when we are captivated by a good book, movie, or project; this happens specifically during those moments when we are so focused that we lose all track of time, food, and the outside world. PEA is noticeably abundant in the brains of happy people.

PEA has also been dubbed the "love chemical." It helps to create feelings of attraction, excitement, and euphoria. When we fall in love our PEA levels increase; we become peppy and full of optimism. The brain releases PEA when we are sexually aroused. PEA levels can peak during orgasm.

When the brain is flooded with PEA, the neurotransmitter dopamine is then blocked from being deactivated and dopamine levels rise. Elevated dopamine levels are associated with increasing mental concentration and a positive attitude.

PEA also increases the effectiveness of another neurotransmitter, norepinephrine, which increases feelings of joy.

In one experiment, investigators found that aerobic exercise can elevate the body's levels of (PEA). PEA is part of the endorphin-induced "runner's high" that enhances energy, mood, and attention. When

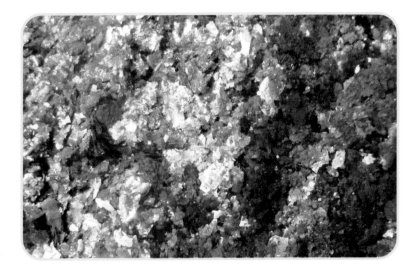

researchers had twenty healthy young men run on a treadmill for 30 minutes, they found that the average concentration of PEA in the participants' urine increased by 77 percent. In addition, the research indicated that patients suffering from depression and bipolar disorder had lower-than-normal levels of PEA in their urine.

PEA is found premade and in great natural abundance in two foods that we know: cacao and blue-green algae (especially in blue phycocyanin). These two foods can significantly elevate the presence of PEA in our brain.

AFA and cacao keep our PEA levels high, no matter what is happening in our life. Blue-green algae works synergistically with cacao in creating a strong ability to focus and pay attention even if we suffer from Attention Deficit Disorder (ADD). One study looking at blue-green algae as a brain food followed 109 students who were fed blue-green algae. The study concluded that the children had a significant improvement in the ability to focus, follow directions, and concentrate. In addition the children experienced a reduction in argumentative, demanding, and combative behavior, fewer symptoms of anxiety and depression, an improvement in social skills, and fewer signs of emotional and behavioral withdrawal.

Drapeau references a study in *Primordial Food* that indicates oral doses of PEA at the rate of 10 mg per day decreased symptoms of depression in 60 percent of the patients tested. In addition, PEA did not cause the patients to gain weight, as most people do with antidepressants; instead, they actually lost weight. AFA contains approximately 2 mg per gram of PEA. AFA concentrates are now available that contain 10 mg of PEA per gram. PEA has no side effects; chemical dependency issues and tolerance limits over time (i.e., doses may stay the same over long periods) are not a concern.

PEA appears to be the primary active ingredient that inhibits appetite and helps people to lose weight when they consume AFA blue-green algae. In a double-blind crossover study involving human patients, supplementing the diets of obese outpatients with 2.8 grams of blue-green algae three times daily over a four-week period resulted in a statistically significant reduction of body weight.

Iron

AFA algae is exceptionally rich in bioavailable iron. When one switches to a vegetarian diet, the iron normally acquired from blood sources (meat) must be drawn from plants, which may be challenging to some individuals. This is where AFA algae can help. AFA is an exceptional source of iron, which works with AFA's manganese, copper, B vitamins, and vitamin C to fight anemia especially in vegetarians who are adapting to non-blood (nonheme) iron sources in plants.

DNA and RNA

DNA and RNA are raw genetic material we call nucleic acids. AFA algae contains approximately 4 percent DNA and RNA. These nucleotides have antimicrobial, antiviral, and antifungal properties. Raw DNA and RNA from AFA algae can be stripped out of the algae by our digestive system and used to assemble new, genetically healthy cells as well as to rejuvenate damaged cells and tissues.

Digestive Wellness

There are thousands of enzymes present in living and/or low-temperature dried AFA algae. These enzymes help to assist our "enzyme cascade," which begins in digestion, continues through the assimilation of nutrients, and ends in metabolism. The more enzymes we have in our diet, the easier time the body has with digestion and metabolism. Raw algae, honey, and grasses (e.g., wheatgrass juice) are some of the richest sources of enzymes.

Antioxidants

We have included a graph comparing the ORAC values of fruits and vegetables with whole AFA super blue-green algae. AFA contains 128 ORAC units per gram.

Beta-Carotene

AFA algae is extraordinarily rich in carotenoids such as beta-carotene. Research continues to demonstrate that the greater the beta-carotene content of one's diet, the longer one lives (as referenced in the spirulina chapter). Research science has shown that beta-carotene activates the thymus gland and the immune system. Dr. Charles Simone, author of *Cancer and Nutrition,* describes that beta-carotene blocks the process whereby healthy cells turn into cancerous cells.

Beta-carotene is one of the safest food nutrients and is nontoxic, even in megadoses. If one's skin begins to turn orange from an extremely high intake of beta-carotene, this is still safe and is not a cause for alarm. It simply indicates that one lacks a liver enzyme that breaks down certain carotene pigments. Some people have this liver enzyme and some people do not have it. If one slows or stops a high intake of carotene, the orange skin color will eventually return to normal.

Fortifying the Immune System

In *Primordial Food,* Drapeau cites research performed by a team of scientists affiliated with the University of Illinois. The team was composed of one board-certified forensic examiner and microbiologist, one surgeon, and three physicians. More than two hundred cases were reviewed in this study. The study concluded that AFA appears to be effective in treating various viral conditions, chronic fatigue, Attention Deficit Disorder (ADD), depression, inflammatory diseases, and fibromyalgia. The study

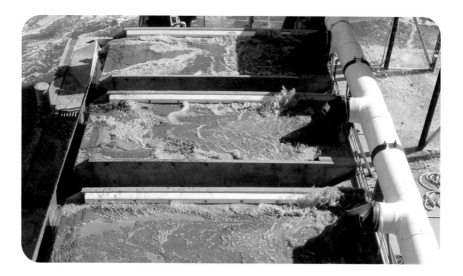

suggests that AFA acts on the immune and nervous systems and prevents inflammation.

Studies done on AFA have demonstrated that it stimulates the migration of stem cells from the bone marrow into the blood and brain (mostly due to the actions of the blue pigment phycocyanin), stimulates white blood cells, and inhibits COX-2 activity, preventing inflammation and improving nervous-system health, as well as one's overall mood.

Drapeau also cites research indicating that AFA, when consumed daily for several weeks, helps move natural killer (NK) cells out of the blood and into the tissues to patrol for and destroy damaged and diseased cells. Although green tea and ginkgo biloba leaf improve the activity of NK cells, no other substance has been found that stimulates this patrolling work.

Researchers have discovered that a blue-green algae protein reduces the ability of the human immunodeficiency virus (HIV) and Ebola virus. The antiviral protein, known as cyanovirin-N (CV-N), can extend the survival time of Ebola-infected mice. There is currently no treatment for Ebola infection, which causes severe and often fatal hemorrhagic fever. "CV-N is extremely effective against a broad range of HIV strains," said Barry O'Keefe, PhD, of NCI's Center for Cancer Research, one of the authors of the study. "CV-N is the first molecule known to inhibit Ebola infection by interfering with the virus's ability to enter cells."

CV-N inhibits HIV and Ebola infection by binding to the outside of the virus and physically blocking it from entering healthy cells. The protein attaches to a particular sugar molecule on the virus surface.

Omega-3 Fatty Acids

AFA contains alpha-linolenic acid (ALA) and the long-chain omega-3 fatty acid known as docosahexanoic acid (DHA). Nearly 50 percent of the fat (oil) content of AFA is composed of these omega-3 essential fatty acids.

In general, most diets worldwide are deficient in omega-3 fatty acids and excessive in omega-6 fatty acids and rancid trans-fatty acids. An excess of omega-6 fatty acids and trans-fats leads to an inflammatory response in the body, which eventually develops into a contributing factor in cardiovascular disease, immunity challenges, neurological problems, and skin disorders.

Omega-3 fatty acids such as ALA and DHA support immunity by help-ing to attract immune cells to the sites of injury, chronic pain, and cellu-lar damage while calming the inflammatory response.

Humans manufacture only small amounts of DHA internally through the consumption of alpha-linolenic acid (ALA), an omega-3 fatty acid commonly found in hempseed, chia, flax, as well as other seeds. This amount of DHA is usually not enough to meet the demands of our nerv-ous system, especially in a high-stress environment.

Traditionally, DHA was acquired directly from eating seafood and fish. With the onset of more seafood allergies and the problems of mercury and PCBs polluting fish, safer forms of DHA have been discovered in other foods. AFA is one of those foods.

DHA is a critical essential fatty acid used in the production and main-tenance of healthy eyesight (retina), brain and nervous system tissue, car-diovascular "slipperiness," and sperm. Long-chain omega-3 fatty acids such as DHA make our cardiovascular system too slippery for calcium-forming nanobacteria (microscopic barnacles) to attach and begin to cal-cify the arteries causing arteriosclerosis.

A deficiency of DHA has been correlated to ADD symptoms, Alzheimer's, arthritis, autoimmune conditions, cardiovascular disease, depression, low brain serotonin levels, neuroses, postpartum depression, and skin disorders.

The therapeutic consumption of omega-3 fatty acids has been shown to improve one's mood and cardiovascular conditions. The consumption of omega-3 also inhibits the formation of breast, colon, pancreatic, and prostate cancer.

AFA Is Nontoxic

During seasonal algal blooms in Klamath Lake, the pH of the water can reach eleven and the oxygen can drop below three parts per million, which can be deadly to fish in the immediate vicinity of the bloom. The death of the fish is not due to any toxins.

Reports that AFA contains toxic proteins have proven to be incorrect. Not only have hundreds of thousands, if not millions, of individuals con-sumed AFA with relatively few cases of side effects, scientific research has indicated that AFA is clear of toxins and that the toxicity of other algae forms may be the source of the confusion.

Some scientists have suggested that AFA blue-green algae contains the amino-acid compound known as β-methylamino alanine (BMAA), and that this amino-acid compound could be linked to neurological problems. Subsequent test results indicated that AFA is devoid of the controversial amino-acid compound known as BMAA.

In *Primordial Food*, Drapeau reports, "In Klamath Lake, nearly ten years of intense testing has failed to reveal the presence of any neurotoxins in its AFA. In 1998, the opinion among scientists was that AFA did not contain neurotoxins and that the original samples that had been identified as AFA were likely another species." He goes on to cite a Wright State University study examining algae genetics that indicated the samples of algae believed to be toxic were not AFA but in fact belonged to the *Anabaena* genera.

As with any superfood or food, people's metabolisms and body chemistry respond to some better than others. I've presented many superfoods in this book so that you can find those that you enjoy the most and that best resonate with your digestion and metabolism.

What to Look For...

AFA Blue-Green Algae Product Types

Below is a list of AFA algae products to look for on the Internet or in your health food store or supplement shop. For years, dried AFA algae products dominated the market. Of the dried AFA algae products, the Refractance Window drying technology methods are considered the best; look for this designation on product labels. In recent years, the company E3Live has made fresh-living liquid AFA algae available as well as other unique AFA formulas and products.

Dried, powdered AFA blue-green algae
E3Live™ Fresh Liquid Algae
AFA blue-green algae chocolate bars and energy bars

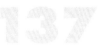
Phycocyanin concentrates (blue pigments of AFA)

PEA concentrates (made from AFA)

AFA blue-green algae probiotics (AFA with friendly digestive bacteria)

How to Use AFA Blue-Green Algae

AFA blue-green algae can cause a detoxification reaction if consumed in too large a quantity initially. Please start yourself and your family on small doses and gradually build up to larger doses over a period of several months.

Recommended Dosages

- Beginner or Child (ages 2–9): 1–2 grams a day (1–2 tsp.)
- Normal or Child (ages 10–18): 2–4 grams a day (2–4 tsp.)
- Therapeutic dose: 8–10 grams a day (8–10 tsp.)
- Super-Athlete dose: as much as 8–12 grams a day (8–12 tsp.)

Simply add the AFA algae to your water, smoothie, shake, or favorite beverage, stir, and drink!

Blue-Green Algae Recipes

Note on all recipes: Three tablespoons of fresh E3Live™ AFA blue-green algae is equivalent to one tablespoon of dried AFA blue-green algae. Special thanks to the SacredChocolate.com staff and the E3Live™ staff for many of the recipe ideas.

Phyto Dressing

1 tbsp. dried AFA

1/3 tbsp. dried marine phytoplankton

4 tbsp. virgin, stone-crushed, organic, olive oil, hempseed oil, or any good quality oil

1/2 tbsp. maca root

1 tsp. organic coconut vinegar or raw apple cider vinegar

2 inches burdock root, chopped and diced

1 small handful of fresh nettles or 2 tbsp. dried nettles

1 pinch of cayenne

1 pinch of turmeric (optional)

Blend all in a blender. Add water to thin the consistency, depending on how thick you want the final dressing. This salad dressing can super-charge your salad. This is a great dressing for athletes interested in building muscle as well as strengthening bones and tendons. It is also great for creating beautiful skin. Tastes great! Enjoy!

E3Live™ Salsa

5 large ripe, red tomatoes, chopped coarse or fine

3 tbsp. finely chopped cilantro

1–2 jalapeno chilies, deseeded and minced

2 cloves finely minced garlic

1 small purple or white onion, finely chopped

2 tsp. lime juice

1–2 pinches Himalayan sea salt or Celtic sea salt (optional)

1 avocado, finely diced (optional)

1 tbsp. E3Live™ fresh liquid, or 2–4 capsules of E3AFA™, or 1–2 tsp. of E3AFA™ Crystal Flakes

Combine all ingredients in a bowl and mix well. Makes about 4 1/2 cups. Serves approximately 8.

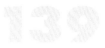
Raw E3Live™ Coconut Chewies

   3 cups of shredded dry coconut

   1 cup raw macadamia nuts or raw cashews

   1 lemon

   1 vanilla bean (just the scraped interior of the bean)

   1/2 cup cacao nibs (optional)

   E3AFA™ dried algae flakes

Place the soaked nuts in the blender and cover with water for one hour. Do not remove water. After one hour, add the peeled lemon (seeds removed) and blend together with water and vanilla on high speed until it's a thick creamy consistency. Add more water if necessary.

Pour nut-and-lemon mixture over shredded dry coconut (and cacao nibs to add a little crunch, if you like) and mix well. Drop by spoonfuls onto the dehydrator sheet and place a generous amount of E3AFA™ dried flakes on top of each cookie. Dehydrate cookies at 105 degrees until thoroughly dried.

Microalgae Super Smoothie

   1–3 tbsp. E3Live™ fresh liquid or 2–4 tsp. of E3AFA™ Crystal Flakes

   1/4 cup strawberries

   1/4 cup blueberries

   1–2 tbsp. spirulina

   1 tsp. chlorella powder

   1 tbsp. powdered marine phytoplankton

   2 tbsp. raw cacao powder

   2 tbsp. of honey

   1/4 cup of pure spring water

Add all ingredients to blender and process until smooth. Excellent when chilled.

Blue-Green Algae Super Smoothie

 2 cups fresh or frozen berries

 1/4 cup cashew nuts

 1/2 avocado

 1 tbsp. hempseed oil

 1/2 gallon (2 liters) of spring water

 3 tbsp. E3Live™ fresh liquid algae

 1 tbsp. dried AFA algae

 1–2 tsp. of E3AFA™ Crystal Flakes

 1 tsp. phycocyanin (blue pigment of AFA algae)

 1 tbsp. fresh bee pollen

Place all ingredients in blender and mix thoroughly until the cashews are completely blended. This powerful smoothie is a dynamic meal replacement. Excellent when chilled.

E3Live™ Vegetable Smoothie

 1/2 cup tomatoes

 1/4 cup chopped red bell pepper

 1/4 cup peeled and chopped cucumber

 1 1/2 tbsp. lemon juice

 1/2 tbsp. chopped scallions

 1/8 tbsp. Celtic sea salt

 1/8 tbsp. fresh-ground pepper

 1–3 tbsp. fresh E3Live™ fresh liquid AFA algae

OPTIONAL:

 1 small slice of fresh habanero or jalapeño pepper

Add all ingredients to a blender and process until smooth.

Blue-Green Algae Green Miracle Soup

1/2 cup tomatoes

1/4 cup chopped red bell pepper

1/4 cup peeled and chopped cucumber

1/3 cup pumpkin seeds

3–5 strips of dulse seaweed

3 stalks dinosaur kale

2 sprigs parsley

1 tbsp. peeled lemon

1/4 onion

1/8 tbsp. Celtic sea salt or Himalayan salt

1/8 tbsp. fresh ground pepper (optional)

1/8 tbsp. hot peppers of any kind

1–3 tbsp. AFA blue-green algae (dried)

1–2 tbsp. green powdered superfoods (select your favorite brand containing superfoods, superherbs, vegetables, grasses, seaweeds, etc.)

Dice and chop the tomatoes, peppers, cucumber, onion, kale, parsley, and lemon into small enough pieces so that all the ingredients will blend smoothly. Add all ingredients to blender and process until smooth.

Warm Blue-Green Algae Elixir

Make an herbal superherb tea containing:

    10 grams pau d'arco

    3.5 grams cat's claw

    2 grams chuchuhuasi

    2 grams chancapiedra

    5 grams goji berries

    1 diced vanilla bean

This will make a half-gallon (2 liters) of tea. Use spring water to make your tea. Bring the superherbs to a scalding temperature, but do not boil. Let steep for an hour, and pour 4 cups of the tea into a blender with the other ingredients:

    1 tbsp. coconut oil

    1 tbsp. raw honey

    1 handful of cacao nibs

    1–3 tbsp. AFA blue-green algae

    1 pinch of Celtic sea salt or Himalayan salt

Blend well. If desired, add your favorite fruits (preferably berries like goji), green superfoods, and supplements. Such optional ingredients may include mesquite powder, soaked Irish moss, ho shou wu (fo-ti), cacao powder, SunWarrior rice protein powder, or tocotrienols.

Stem Cell Immune Illume Elixir

1/2 liter spring water

1/4 cup lemon juice

1/4 cup blueberries (preferably wild)

1–2 tsp. camu camu berry powder

1–2 tbsp. noni powder

1–3 tbsp. E3Live™ fresh liquid algae

1–2 tsp. of E3AFA™ crystal flakes

2 tbsp. phycocyanin (blue pigments of AFA algae)

500–1000 mg reishi mushroom mycelium powder

500–1000 mg maitake mushroom mycelium powder

2–4 grams sacha jergon superherb powder

2–4 capsules of MegaHydrate™

1/4 cup goji berries (optional)

2 tbsp. of honey (optional)

Add all the ingredients to the blender and blend into a tonic elixir. Add more spring water if necessary. This elixir taken daily will seriously ramp up one's immune system. Do not add honey or goji berries if you are fighting candida or cancer. Sweet foods of all kinds should be avoided as much as possible when dealing with candida or cancer.

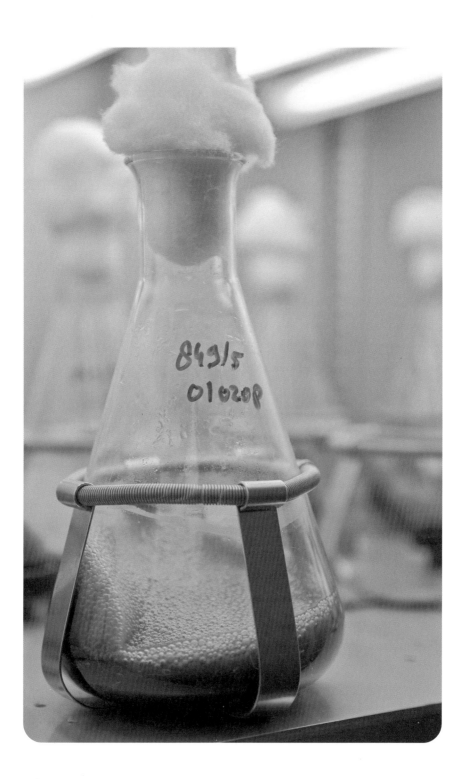

Marine Phytoplankton

The Basis of All Life

The sea, the great unifier, is man's only hope. Now, as never before, the old phrase has a literal meaning: we are all in the same boat.

—Jacques-Yves Cousteau

Latin Names:

Major varieties: *Nannochloropsis*

Common Names:

Marine phytoplankton, phytoplankton, plankton, microalgae, *Worfuhlun*

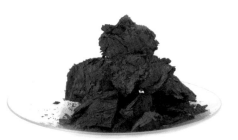

Superfood Type:

Green phytoplankton (liquid, powder, paste)

History, Facts, and Legends

The future of nutrition is found in the ocean.

—Jacques-Yves Cousteau

My first introduction to marine phytoplankton was a television program hosted by Jacques Cousteau when I was a child. The program featured Cousteau's revelations about "plankton as the basis of the food chain." This was so extraordinary to me because at the time our family lived on the New Jersey shore. I used to ride my bicycle on the boardwalk near the ocean and stare out into the waves, even during the wintertime, imagining all the marine phytoplankton out there.

For an estimated three billion years, marine phytoplankton have directly supported virtually all living creatures in the ocean and, indirectly, all those creatures on land.

There are an estimated forty thousand species of marine phytoplankton and microalgae in the oceans, lakes, rivers, creeks, and waterways of the Earth. Marine phytoplankton make up one quarter of all vegetation (land and sea) and according to NASA provide up to 90 percent of the oxygen in the air we breathe. Marine phytoplankton produce more oxygen than all the Earth's forests combined. Scientific research indicates that marine phytoplankton may be the most important food on planet Earth not only because of the nutritional content of the phytoplankton, but also because marine phytoplankton is food for everything on Earth—these organisms represent the very meaning of food.

Marine phytoplankton also produce more sulfur than all of the world's life-forms combined. Phytoplankton secrete sulfur byproducts known as DMSP and DMS—these compounds are nearly identical to DMSO (dimethyl sulfoxide) and MSM (methyl-sulfonyl-methane), and as they evaporate off the oceans they form clouds above the phytoplankton that protect the phytoplankton, protecting against excessive radiation from the sun. When clouds form, the phytoplankton slow and/or stop their production of sulfur. This closed feedback loop is very likely the basis of the Earth's weather systems. Through ensuing rain this bioavailable sulfur is then spread around the world and distributed to all the land plants and animals. Not only is sulfur spread into the atmosphere and across the land in this way, winds and weather often lift the marine phytoplankton organisms themselves right into the atmosphere. Frozen marine phytoplankton cells have been found in clouds that have drifted over the Great Plains of the United States, far away from the oceans.

In one of the great ironies of the natural world, single-celled marine phytoplankton (the smallest plant organisms on the planet) support and feed the largest animal on the planet—the majestic blue whale. The blue whale is the largest mammal that has ever lived, and can weigh up to two hundred tons. This king of the ocean feeds exclusively on marine phytoplankton and select species of krill (krill eat only phytoplankton). A blue whale can travel hundreds of miles without rest, and consumes up to 1.5 million calories per day in order to meet its enormous energy requirements.

Overall, as a class of creatures, the whales eat a diet consisting mainly of marine phytoplankton, with the exception of the omnivorous whales. Whales produce the largest brains and healthiest nervous systems of any living family of mammals due to their consumption of this superfood. Their life span ranges between eighty and one hundred and fifty years. And, many of them remain sexually active until death.

Marine phytoplankton contain a unique and extraordinary combination of life-sustaining nutrients including omega-3 essential fatty acids (including docosahexaenoic acid or DHA), nucleotides, DNA, RNA, protein, chlorophyll, vitamins, major minerals, trace elements, and polysaccharides.

Of the forty thousand species of microalgae and marine phytoplankton, several dozen of the leading varieties useful to human nutrition are now being grown in various photobioreactor environments.

Photobioreactors

How does one procure marine phytoplankton? Of course, we could go out into the center of the ocean and procure plankton by skimming it off the top layers of the ocean with very thin nets but ship travel, erratic weather, lack of quality controls, contaminants, and poor collection techniques make it extremely challenging to accomplish this task.

On dry land in several places around the world, giant photobioreactors (PBRs) have been constructed to grow marine phytoplankton in a completely controlled environment. Because of the presence of so many other organisms, the open ocean cannot be used to grow a controlled culture of marine phytoplankton. Photobioreactors replicate the natural growing conditions found in the wild ocean, but with the added benefit that one can restrict the exchange of gases and water, as well as completely control contaminants between the culture and the outside environment. PBRs have several advantages over open pond systems for the cultivation of microalgae:

- Higher biomass concentrations
- Eliminated and/or significantly reduced contaminants
- Better control of biological and chemical specifications
- Better control of algal culture
- Large surface-to-volume ratio
- Better control of gas transfer
- Reduction in evaporation of growth medium
- More uniform temperature
- Higher algal cell densities are possible

For some applications, these advantages justify the increased cost of PBRs compared to open ponds. Open ponds are used, for example, to grow spirulina, but they do not provide the conditions necessary for high-density algal biomass production because of the variation in light intensity and temperature throughout the seasons of the year.

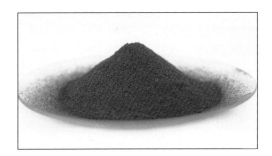

Benefits

The makeup of marine phytoplankton is exactly what human cell membranes need to carry out their metabolism. Research indicates that marine phytoplankton contains every nutrient needed for the creation and maintenance of new cells.

Board-certified family Integrative Medicine practitioner and author Dr. Hugo Rodier comments on marine phytoplankton:

> The problem is that we need ALL of them [nutrients] at the same time for things to work. One of those rare products that contain almost everything you need for life is marine phytoplankton. It contains all nine

amino acids that the body cannot make. The essential fatty acids are also present (omega-3 and omega-6). Vitamins A, B1, B2, B3, B5, B6, B12, C, D, and major trace minerals are all present in phytoplankton.

Since marine phytoplankton is the basis of the Earth's entire food chain, it provides extraordinary nutrition to all life at all ages—it's beneficial for you, your children, your parents, your pets, your trees, your plants, and more. Marine phytoplankton is:

- The best plant-based source of long-chain omega-3 fatty acids (DHA, EPA).
- A natural source of wide-spectrum, plant-based vitamins, minerals, antioxidants, polysaccharides, and protein.
- A complete protein source. In fact, marine phytoplankton—like AFA blue-green algae, spirulina, and chlorella—is over 60 percent protein by weight.

Phytoplankton is 100 percent bioavailable to the human body; when you eat it, not a single part of it is wasted. (This is astounding, because even the healthiest foods contain less than 50 percent absorbable and available nutrition.) The benefits of using marine phytoplankton are:

- *Energy without stimulation:* Solid, consistent energy throughout the day is vital to all of us. Phytoplankton delivers vital life force at the mitochondria level of cellular energy production even though phytoplankton contains no stimulants such as caffeine. Phytoplankton contains the energy currency required by the human body, called nucleotides (ATP, GTP, etc.). Theoretically, if enough of the nucleotide energy units are supplied to a cell, not only does the cell's energy increase, but DNA repair can also occur. I learned about this from the controversial Dr. George Merkl and his work on the "life crystal," which he told me he first isolated in phytoplankton.
- *An improved immune system:* Antiviral, antifungal, and antibacterial effects have been reported as a result of consuming marine phytoplankton.
- *Aches and pains decrease:* Anti-inflammatory effects have been observed with phytoplankton use. Because of its nucleotide content and effect in increasing cellular and immune system energy without stimulation,

marine phytoplankton may be capable of driving back inflammatory infections.

- *Improved speed and safety of detoxification:* The high-alkaline mineral and energy content of marine phytoplankton makes it an ideal detoxification tool. You can take phytoplankton daily while cleansing and/or fasting. Phytoplankton facilitates detoxification without demineralization. Herbal cleansing systems and fasting are helpful for detoxification, but can also cause demineralization (loss of minerals in the metabolism, tissue, or bones). Important minerals such as calcium, magnesium, sulfur, and zinc help protect the body and guide toxins out. If these minerals are not provided for in the diet, they will be drawn out of the bones and vital organs, causing demineralization. Superfoods in general, and marine phytoplankton in particular, solve this problem.

- *Lose weight:* Marine phytoplankton helps shed excess weight and fat effortlessly because you will be getting dozens of known (and some unknown) minerals in each drop or teaspoon of powder, as well as thousands of other nutrients.

- *Improved memory:* Your memory and brainpower can improve. Marine phytoplankton contain the smallest nanoparticulate size of all microalgae and several of its nutrients, including the phospholipids and omega-3 fatty acids, are able to cross the blood-brain barrier feeding the brain and master glands located deep in the brain, which stimulates significant neurotransmitter production as well as mental clarity.

- *Feeling stronger and more athletic:* The intense chlorophyll content in phytoplankton also increases oxygen uptake. Higher oxygen uptake means more fuel to muscles, which translates to improved performance and endurance. In addition, phytoplankton is a complete protein source. Because this superfood protein is typically uncooked, it is twice as absorbable as cooked protein.

- *Normalizing blood sugar imbalances:* Blood sugar disorders (mineral deficiency syndromes) will naturally decrease in their severity. More balance will be achieved with the restoration of the much-needed minerals that healthy, healing phytoplankton products can provide.

- *Fewer cravings:* Gradually you will begin to naturally stop craving unhealthy, processed, mineral-deficient food due to the restoration of the mineral profile of each organ in your body. All superfoods are effective at helping to heal cravings.

- *Improved concentration:* Due to a heightened level of brain nutrition, concentration will improve so you can get more done in less time. This means more free time with family, friends, and creative pursuits.
- *Better sex:* With more energy and improved physical systems you will enjoy better sex.
- *Faster recovery:* You will recover from illness and/or injury more quickly due to the cumulative effect of improved cellular repair.
- *Nervous system repair:* Marine phytoplankton is a useful tool against chronic neurological challenges. Advanced nutrition research indicates that marine phytoplankton products contain nervous-system repair factors such as phospholipids, DHA, and EPA that help repair damaged myelin sheathing (the protective layer around each nerve fiber).
- *Calm and well-being:* If you practice meditation, you will find your mind calmer and your body easier to calm down. Overall, a residual "grounding energy" will be felt.
- *Better sleep:* You will find it easier to go to sleep and to sleep restfully all night long.
- *More energy to start your day:* You will awaken more refreshed and ready to tackle the day.
- *Improved digestion and circulation:* This is due to the concentration of minerals and chlorophyll in marine phytoplankton.
- *Improved eyesight:* This is likely because the extraordinary antioxidant content of phytoplankton as well as the presence of long-chain omega-3 fatty acids (DHA, EPA) directly nourish the eyes.
- *Feeling younger:* The rich mineral content of marine phytoplankton will make your skin appear more vibrant and younger because minerals such as zinc, sulfur, and silicon act as inner cosmetics that naturally beautify skin cells.

People who include marine phytoplankton in their diet are known to enjoy enhanced brain function, improved immune function, antiviral/antifungal/antibacterial effects, improved cellular repair, radiation protection, detoxification support, anti-inflammatory support, antioxidant support, improved circulation, improved heart function, allergy/asthma relief, suppression of symptoms stemming from degenerative disease, and a residual "grounding energy" overall. There are hundreds of references in scientific journals detailing the vast array of health benefits gained through the consumption of marine phytoplankton and microalgae such as spirulina, AFA blue-green algae, and chlorella.

Mike Adams, chief editor of www.naturalnews.com, stated in an article on marine phytoplankton that phytoplankton is beneficial in helping improve the following conditions:

Rheumatoid arthritis
Type-2 diabetes
Autoimmune disorders such as lupus
Eczema and skin disorders
Breast cancer, prostate cancer, and other cancers
Heart disease and atherosclerosis
Alzheimer's disease and dementia
Chronic fatigue syndrome
Parkinson's disease and other neuromuscular disorders
Liver disease and hepatitis
Depression, mood swings, and behavioral disorders
Eye disease
Infertility and reproductive system disorders
Infections and common colds
Asthma and respiratory disorders
Kidney and bladder disorders
Osteoporosis and skeletal disorders
Chronic pain and joint pain

Gram for gram, marine phytoplankton is likely the most nutrient-dense, alkaline superfood on Earth. This is a superfood that contains all known minerals, all known amino acids—almost everything you could name that could be potentially missing in our nutrition!

Improve Omega-3 Fatty Acid Absorption

Omega-3 fats are essential to human health. Continuing research has demonstrated that the consumption of omega-3 fatty acids leads to a reduced risk in developing cardiovascular disease, autoimmune disorders, neurological problems, and behavioral disorders. The better the absorption of omega-3 fatty acids into the brain and nervous system, the more efficient and swift will be the healing results.

In general, marine phytoplankton is superior to fish oil as a source for phospholipids that help us absorb long-chain, omega-3 fatty acids. It is these phospholipids that should be taken with fish, krill, and/or algae oils to make the fish and algae oils more effective in reaching the brain, nervous system, and eyes. In essence, the efficacy of fish oils, including cod liver oil, krill, and algae oils, will be improved when taken with marine phytoplankton. Not only that, like fish, krill, and some algae oils, marine phytoplankton contain one or both of the key omega-3 fatty acids: docosahexaenoic acid (DHA) and eicosapentaenoic acid (EPA). Therefore, not only is marine phytoplankton helping to potentiate omega-3 fatty acids, it also contains them.

If you are a strict vegan or vegetarian and do not choose to consume any animal products whatsoever, then marine phytoplankton is strongly recommended. This will supply you with the essential long-chain forms of omega-3 (DHA and EPA). Importantly, these forms of omega-3 fatty acids are different from the medium-chain omega-3 alpha-linolenic acid (ALA) found in flax oil and hempseed oil. ALA may or may not be converted by the human body into the more needed long-chain DHA and EPA. This conversion depends on numerous factors, including the presence of B vitamins, minerals such as magnesium, the presence of phospholipids, the presence of coconut oil, and metabolic factors in each individual's biology. Marine phytoplankton's phospholipids, B vitamins, and minerals help convert ALA to DHA and EPA. Marine phytoplankton itself also contains ALA.

Phospholipids are needed to transport fat-soluble nutrients into our system and then, potentially, into our brain. The ALA-, DHA- and EPA-bearing oils, when taken with the phytoplankton, can more easily cross the blood-brain barrier into the brain. This blood-brain barrier protects the brain from most foreign substances blocking their entry. In essence, the transfer mechanism to the brain (where we need ALA, DHA, and EPA the most) is more efficient with phytoplankton.

ATP and Energy

With the smallest nanoparticulate size of all microalgae, marine phytoplankton delivers vital life energy at the DNA and mitochondria level and also penetrates the blood-brain barrier, feeding the higher master glands located deep in the brain and stimulating significant mental clarity.

Normally our bodies have to break down everything we eat into little packets of protein, sugar, fats, and oils, which are put into one end of the mitochondria factory, and come out the other side as tiny energy units called nucleotides (ATP, ADP, AGP, etc.). These nucleotides are the currency of the cell—the biological battery packets that are used to produce cellular energy. The nucleotides in phytoplankton actually bypass the mitochondria production factory altogether because phytoplankton nucleotides directly feed the cell with energy. This means that the cell can produce energy quickly and effectively without having to go through all the energy of digestion.

Marine phytoplankton products also help to produce cellular energy without containing any significant calories because they bypass the mitochondria (the energy powerhouses of the cell). Taking medium-to-high doses of marine phytoplankton produces energy with no stimulation. The ATP and other nucleotides turn directly into energy once in the human body, which makes marine phytoplankton the leading superfood product in the world for those needing to work extra hard in high-stress environments without sleep and who require long-term energy and focus without stimulants. In this department, marine phytoplankton is unsurpassed.

Antioxidants

Marine phytoplankton is rich in antioxidants such as chlorophyll as well as rejuvenating, immunizing, and cancer-fighting carotenoids including yellow- and red-pigmented xanthophylls.

Chlorophyll is one of the planet's most widely utilized antioxidants. Antioxidants protect us from excessive radiation including x-ray screening at airports, ultraviolet rays from the sun, radioactive debris in the atmosphere and in the food supply (depleted uranium), reactive oxygen (free radicals), airplane travel, chemtrails, and more.

The intense chlorophyll content in marine phytoplankton also increases oxygen uptake, which means more fuel to the muscles for improved performance and endurance.

What to Look For...

Marine Phytoplankton Types

Powdered marine phytoplankton: Teams of doctors, microbiologists, scientists and botanists from around the world have spent many years and billions of dollars researching the forty thousand species of marine phytoplankton to determine the best species in each category to use for biofuel, aquaculture, exotic fish food, and ultimately, human consumption.

As a result of this extensive research, technologically advanced commercial facilities have now been constructed to produce pure, uncontaminated marine phytoplankton in large volume using sophisticated photobioreactors (PBRs). PBRs consist of extensive tubing interconnected in a horizontal grid the size of a football field. A "spring plankton bloom" environment is created that allows natural photosynthesis to occur, using sunlight to grow the marine phytoplankton biomass. The purified seawater solution in which the marine phytoplankton grows ensures that there are no other species contaminating the biomass. This method produces a pure, "beyond organic" super-concentrated biomass of phytoplankton. Essentially, PBRs create a controlled, chemical-free environment that makes the end phytoplankton product consistently free from environmental contaminants. Not all marine phytoplankton products are produced in this way, some are still naturally harvested from the wild ocean.

Approximately 200 species of marine phytoplankton were found to be beneficial for human consumption. Several edible species of marine phytoplankton are now being sold as powdered, dried superfood products, with new ones entering the market all the time. They have a powdered consistency similar to spirulina. In my household we consider powdered marine phytoplankton an essential component of our powdered superfood collection, in which all items are ready to include in superfood smoothies, concoctions, elixirs, and treats.

Liquid marine phytoplankton: These products are available in dropper bottles. They are not as concentrated and nutritious as powdered phytoplankton products. Their primary benefit is ease of use.

Bottled beverages containing marine phytoplankton: Several companies offer combination beverages of superfoods and herbs with marine phytoplankton added. These companies have done a tremendous job of educating people about the power of marine phytoplankton.

How to Use Marine Phytoplankton

Like all the other superfoods, marine phytoplankton is highly concentrated compared to most other human foods, so only a relatively small quantity is required in order to achieve useful health benefits.

Liquid or dried marine phytoplankton may be added to spring water, superfood smoothies, fresh juices, elixirs, and raw chocolate (cacao) concoctions or, in the case of prepared phytoplankton beverages, it can be consumed as delivered. Consume marine phytoplankton with "hyper oils" such as fish oil, krill oil, or vegan-friendly algae oil, or with coconut oil for enhanced effects. Using Dr. Patrick Flanagan's MegaHydrate™ super-antioxidant product along with both the marine phytoplankton and any of these oils is extremely effective in enhancing the rejuvenating effect of all these products on the nervous system.

Due to phytoplankton's natural biological relationship with sulfur, I recommend that you also try using MSM (methyl-sulfonyl-methane) powder in your beverage when you add marine phytoplankton. Start with a small amount, a teaspoon for example, and increase from there. This appears to amplify the potency of both products, especially the anti-inflammatory and antioxidant effects.

After experimenting with marine phytoplankton for just a few days, you will notice how powerful the energizing effects of this superfood can be.

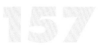
Warning: Marine phytoplankton, like nearly all microalgae, contains significant amounts of vitamin K, which some studies have shown to interfere with blood-thinning medications.

How to Store Marine Phytoplankton

Once your marine phytoplankton product is opened, it should be (but do not have to be) refrigerated in order to maintain maximum freshness. It is recommended that these products be used within three months after opening.

Marine Phytoplankton Recipes

Super Silica and Brain Builder Juice

Recipe by Frank Giglio

> 2 cucumbers
>
> 1/2 lemon-yellow peel removed, white pith intact
>
> 4 celery stalks
>
> 1–2 tsp. marine phytoplankton powder

Using a juicer, juice the cucumber, celery and lemon. Stir in the marine phytoplankton and enjoy. Consider spiking all your vegetable juices with marine phytoplankton!

Marine Maca Superherb Elixir

Follow the tea recipes below. To create the hot tea base, bring the tea ingredients to just below a boil in 1.5 quarts (1.5 liters) of spring water, then turn off heat and allow to steep covered in the pot for 5 minutes.

TEA RECIPE:

Chaga (wild, dried, ping pong ball sized) (superherb from the northern hemisphere's temperate forests)

1 slice of rhodiola (dried root) (adaptogenic superherb)

2 tbsp. nettles (tea cut) (anti-inflammatory superherb)

2 tbsp. horsetail (anti-fungal, bone building superherb)

Add the strained contents of the hot tea base (above) to a blender already containing:

1 tbsp. marine phytoplankton

2 tbsp. maca

2 tbsp. almond butter

1 tbsp. hempseeds

1–2 tbsp. hempseed oil

3 tbsp. NoniLand™ honey (or other favorite raw honey)

1–2 tbsp. of medicinal mushroom powders containing (reishi, maitake, lion's mane, cordyceps)

1 pinch cayenne pepper (to taste)

Blend until completely creamy and frothy. This drink allows you to survive arctic conditions with superhero resilience! Brave cold weather with ease! Enjoy.

Serves three.

Spiked Up Orange Juice

Recipe by Frank Giglio

>   12 ounces fresh squeezed orange juice
>
>   1–2 tsp. camu camu berry powder
>
>   1 squirt of Crystal Energy
>
>   1–2 tsp. marine phytoplankton powder
>
>   1 dropper Super Ionic Minerals
>
>   1/4 tsp. cayenne pepper (optional)

Blend or shake all the ingredients together. This drink is perfect to energize the body or add a little warmth when "under the weather."

Spring Water, Honey, Plankton Cocktail

>   1 quart (liter) spring water
>
>   1–2 tsp. powdered marine phytoplankton
>
>   2 tbsp. raw honey
>
>   1–2 pinches Celtic sea salt or Himalayan salt

Blend or shake all the ingredients together. This is a phenomenal energy drink for long hikes on hot days.

Chunky Marine Avocado Salsa

Recipe by Frank Giglio

    2 medium sized ripe avocados, cut into chunks

    1/4 cup red onion, minced

    1 small clove garlic, minced

    juice of 1 lime

    1/4 cup fresh cilantro, roughly chopped

    1–2 tsp. marine phytoplankton powder

    1–2 small chili peppers (optional)

    1 head of bib lettuce or romaine

Add all ingredients, except lettuce to a mixing bowl. Gently stir them together. Season to taste with sea salt. Add optional chili pepper. Once the desired flavor is reached, spoon small quantities onto the lettuce. Serve and enjoy.

Super Brain, Eye, and Nervous System Rejuvenation Drink

water and flesh from 2 coconuts or 1/2 liter of spring water

2 heaping tbsp. coconut oil

1–2 tsp. freeze-dried powdered marine phytoplankton

1200 mg. (3–4 gel caps) krill oil, fish oil, and/or algae oil

2–4 capsules Dr. Patrick Flanagan's MegaHydrate™

1000 mg. (2 vegetable capsules) lion's mane mushroom (powder)

2 tbsp. raw honey

1 cup blueberries (preferably fresh, although frozen is fine)

1 cup raspberries (preferably fresh, although frozen is fine)

Open the two coconuts and pour out the water into a blender. Spoon the coconut meat out and put in the blender. If you have no coconuts, use fresh spring water. The MegaHydrate™ and lion's mane may be encapsulated; open the desired milligram amount of capsules and pour the powder into the blender. If the oils are in gelatin capsules, poke a hole in the oil gel capsules and squeeze the desired milligram dosage into the blender. Add the remaining ingredients. Blend and enjoy.

This drink has the power to rejuvenate difficult-to-reach nerve tissue. It improves eyesight, memory, and helps alleviate neurological problems. The coconut oil, marine phytoplankton, and MegaHydrate™ help improve the absorption of omega-3 fatty acids.

Marine Phytoplankton Sulfur Electrolyte Lemonade

- 1 quart (liter) spring water
- 1 handful goji berries
- 1–2 tsp. powdered marine phytoplankton
- 1 whole skinned lemon with the seeds removed
- 2 tbsp. MSM powder
- 2 tbsp. raw NoniLand™ honey or Manuka honey
- 2–3 pinches Celtic sea salt
- 1 squirt Dr. Patrick Flanagan's Crystal Energy

Place all ingredients in a blender. Blend briefly. Serve chilled. This beverage is excellent for blood-rejuvenating electrolytes and for tissue hydration. The sulfur (MSM), electrolytes, and trace minerals also improve the skin, hair, and nails.

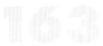

Ormus Phytoplankton Happy Electrolyte Lemonade

   1 quart (liter) spring water

   1–2 tsp. powdered marine phytoplankton

   1 whole skinned lemon with the seeds removed

   2 droppersful of David Wolfe's Ormus Gold

   2 tbsp. raw NoniLand™ honey or Manuka honey

   2–3 pinches Celtic sea salt

   1 squirt Dr. Patrick Flanagan's Crystal Energy

Place all ingredients in a blender. Blend briefly. Serve chilled. This beverage is excellent for providing blood-rejuvenating electrolytes, tissue hydration, and digestive system rejuvenation. The Ormus Gold helps stimulate serotonin and the "feel good" neurotransmitters.

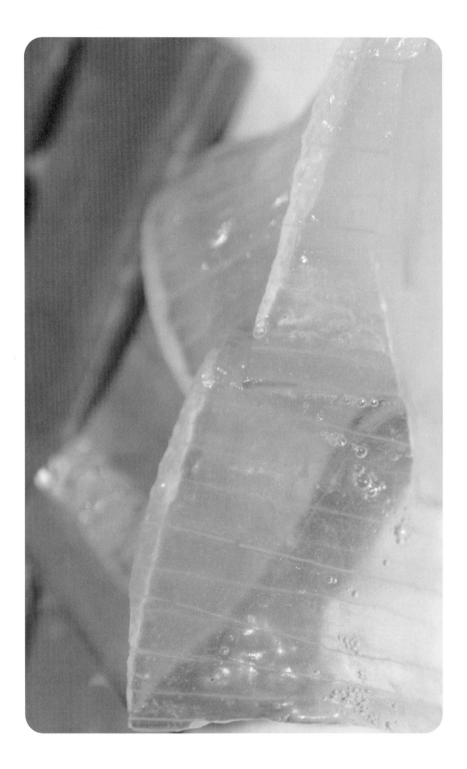

Aloe Vera

Essene and Egyptian Secret of Immortality

Latin Names:

Aloe barbadensis

Aloe ferox

Common Names:

Aloe Vera, Aloe, Burn Plant, Sa'vila (Spanish), Ghrita-kumari (Sanskrit), Jadam (Malaysian), Lu-hui (Chinese), Erva babosa (Portuguese)

Superfood Type:

Leaf

History, Facts, and Legends

Later, Joseph of Arimathea asked Pilate for the body of Jesus. Now Joseph was a disciple of Jesus, but secretly, because he feared the Jews. With Pilate's permission, he came and took the body away. He was accompanied by Nicodemus, the man who earlier had visited Jesus at night. Nicodemus brought a mixture of myrrh and aloes, about seventy-five pounds. Taking Jesus' body, the two of them wrapped it, with the spices, in strips of linen. This was in accordance with Jewish burial customs. At the place where Jesus was crucified, there was a garden, and in the garden a new tomb, in which no one had ever been laid. Because it was

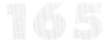

the Jewish day of Preparation and since the tomb was nearby, they laid Jesus there.

—John 19:38–42

The aloe genus contains over two hundred species that grow across the desert and subtropical regions of Africa, America, Asia, and Europe. The primary aloe vera varieties we know are a desert succulent native to Africa which is now grown all over the world. A member of the lily family, aloe vera is one of the most nutritious vegetables on the planet. Each leaf of fresh aloe vera contains a mucilaginous gel, which is a potent source of long-chain sugars known as polysaccharides. The thick aloe vera leaves must be "filleted" to remove the gel.

Aloe vera is truly a superfood gift from the ancient Egyptians, who first discovered the magic of this food and bred aloe into most of the cultivars we see today. The rumored secret of Cleopatra's famed beauty and youth continues to point to the obvious—the application of aloe vera to her skin.

The Essenes, a Jewish sect, inherited aloe from the Egyptians and continued to cultivate this impressive plant near the Dead Sea at Qumran. The Essenes ate raw and living foods, smelted metals, experimented with chemistry, and consumed aloe as their primary superfood, which they grew in soil rich with Dead Sea salt extracts. The Roman historian Josephus recorded that the Essenes often lived to be one hundred and twenty-five years of age during a time when the average life span was thirty-nine years.

The Greeks also inherited their knowledge of aloe vera from the Egyptians. Due to the influence of his mentor Aristotle, Alexander the Great was quite fond of aloe vera. His armies carried potted aloe vera with them on military campaigns. Aloe was applied to the wounds of his soldiers. Alexander conquered the island of Socotra in the Indian Ocean in order to procure aloe (Socotra is currently part of the nation of Yemen).

Benefits

The gel of raw aloe vera contains vitamins A, C, and E, the minerals sulfur, calcium, magnesium, zinc, selenium, and chromium, as well as antioxidants, fiber, amino acids, enzymes, sterols, lignins, and, most importantly, polysaccharides.

Aloe's polysaccharides have a particular lubricating effect on the joints, brain, nervous system, and the skin. These polysaccharides are long-burning carbohydrates and provide steady energy over time.

Aloe vera polysaccharides have immuno-modulating effects. They allow the human immune system to fight back chronic viral, nanobacteria, and fungal infections.

Aloe vera is a crucial part of any weight loss and fitness program as it has been shown that when you ingest aloe, you can lose weight and also gain lean muscle mass.

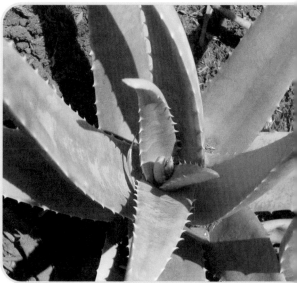

If you want to be beautiful all the days of your life, if you want to be flexible and limber all the days of your life, if you want to have an immune system and nervous system that work well for all the days of your life, aloe vera is the super-food for you.

Creating Digestive Wellness with Aloe's Antimicrobial Properties

Aloe vera is helpful for all types of digestive problems and can aid in recovery from digestive illnesses, such as colitis, ulcers, and irritable bowel syndrome. Research suggests that aloe vera polysaccharides are responsible for the calming effects on digestion. Additionally, aloe's ability to support the replication of healthy epithelial cells that line our inner digestive environment is well known.

Aloe vera cuts and dissolves mucous in the intestines, which helps increase nutrient absorption.

Aloe's mannose polysaccharide is effective at killing yeast (candida). In clinical human research, acemannan (mannose chains) from aloe improved food digestion and absorption and enhanced the presence of friendly bacteria (probiotics such as *acidophilus*) in the digestive tract by reducing yeast and normalizing pH levels. Aloe acts as a prebiotic—this means it potentiates the effectiveness of probiotics such as *acidophilus, bifidus, L. salivarius, L. plantarum,* etc.; it makes them work better.

The polysaccharides in aloe vera are converted by the human body into oligosaccharides, which protect the mucosal lining of the digestive tract and have been shown to be effective in fighting back the following organisms:

> *Bordetella pertussis* (whooping cough pathogen)
> *E. coli strains*
> *Heliobacter pylori*
> *Streptococcus pneumoniae*

Individuals with Crohn's disease have been found to be deficient in oligosaccharides in their digestive system.

Reducing Inflammation, Radiation Sickness, Cancer, Heart Disease, and Diabetes

In studies done on rodents, aloe vera has demonstrated the ability to markedly inhibit arthritis, edema, and inflammation. Aloe also stimulated the production of fibroblasts in rodents, indicating the healing of damaged tissue was occurring. The results specifically indicated a 50 percent reduction in inflammation. Mast cells, which are active in autoimmune and allergic responses, decreased by 48 percent.

Studies have demonstrated that aloe vera reduces radiation sickness in animals. Aloe helped them gain weight and recover faster with less nausea after being exposed to the radiation. Topical treatments using acemannan aloe extract reduced skin reactions in animals to radiation significantly.

A study done in Milan, Italy, on twenty-six patients with advanced solid tumors including cancers of the breast, digestive tract, brain, and lung were treated daily with twenty milligrams of the tryptamine neurotransmitter melatonin. Another twenty-four patients were treated with the twenty milligrams of melatonin along with one milliliter twice a day of an alcohol-based tincture of aloe vera. An improvement occurred in two of the twenty-four patients and fourteen of the patients stabilized and did not experience worse symptoms. Of the twenty-six patients treated with melatonin only, only seven stabilized.

In a five-year study done on five thousand patients with angina pain caused by coronary heart disease, subjects were given the option to consume aloe and a psyllium fiber containing polysaccharides. In those consuming the aloe and psyllium, total serum cholesterol, serum triglycerides, and total lipids were markedly reduced and healthy HDL was increased. The patients who most benefited were diabetics.

The raw gel of fresh aloe vera has been shown to aid in the normalization of blood sugar, helping to lessen the symptoms of diabetes. Recent studies have shown that levels of the important antioxidants vitamins C and E remained elevated for twenty-four hours after taking the fresh gel internally, providing a gentle, time-release effect of these vitamins in the body. Consumption of the fresh gel has also been shown to stimulate the body's own antioxidant defenses and increase the bioavailability of naturally occurring antioxidants found in foods and whole-food supplements.

Ormus, Polysaccharides, and the Immune System

The polysaccharides found in raw, fresh aloe vera are one part of a larger family of essential glyconutrients, long-chain sugars that the body needs in order to maintain a strong immune system and achieve radiant health.

Specifically, aloe vera contains mannose polysaccharides strung together. These mannose clusters are known by different names, including acemannan, acetylated polymannans, polymannose, and APM. Mannose is antibacterial, antifungal, antiviral, and antiparasitic. Mannose reduces inflammation.

Polysaccharides such as those found in raw, fresh aloe vera may also be found in practically every superfood and superherb, yet aloe, noni, and the medicinal mushrooms (reishi, chaga, maitake, shiitake, cordyceps, etc.) lead them all in overall healing polysaccharide content.

Aloe has a high affinity to concentrate Ormus minerals, a type of strange matter or "high energy particles" known to the ancients, but lost in time until rediscovered in the 1970s by alchemist David Radius Hudson in his research on Arizona basalt rock. David Hudson's research indicated that aloe vera concentrates Ormus minerals in the polysaccharide fraction of the aloe's gel.

Polysaccharides carry the Ormus minerals that have an affinity for the surface of our joints, for our nervous and immune systems, our skin and hair, as well as our pancreas and liver. These healing long-chain sugars carrying Ormus have been identified with aloe vera's historical use as an aid to immunity, the digestive system, and the skin. These polysaccharides containing Ormus act as a unifying biological force, modulating the energies of all the biologically active compounds and living cells they contact, leading to accelerated healing and a deep, optimal homeostatic balance.

I have grown aloe vera to perfection in my office by using dilute amounts of pure Dead Sea salt and Dead Sea salt extracts. Dead Sea salt contains the highest concentration of Ormus minerals of any known substance. Using some Dead Sea salt occasionally in one's aloe vera soil mix or diluted in the watering container allows the aloe vera to access more Ormus minerals. One leaf that I broke off a Dead-Sea-salt-grown aloe remained unchanged and "alive" in my kitchen for over three months while I was traveling.

Hydration

Aloe's polysaccharides contain hydrogen and Ormus concentrates that increase the hydration of epithelial cells. Hydrogen is what is needed to create "hydration." In order to remain hydrated one must consume enough hydrogen. In indigenous desert environments where water is scarce, consuming aloe is a crucial part of survival.

The sulfur contained in aloe has been shown to be in forms similar to DMSO (dimethyl sulfoxide) and its important chemical relative MSM (methyl-sulfonyl-methane). These forms of sulfur are effective at hydrating dried-out, leathery tissue (collagen damage, wrinkles, hardening of the organs, etc.), thus restoring juiciness, elasticity, and flexibility. These sulfur forms are also known to help our immune system dissolve nanobacteria that cause hardening in dehydrated tissue. Nanobacteria are virus-sized, shell-forming organisms that cause arthritis, autoimmune disorders, heart disease, cataracts, kidney stones, gall stones, psoriasis, and more.

Aloe's Ormus-carrying polysaccharides can stimulate collagen production, which retains moisture, resulting in younger-looking skin. Ormus compounds have been found to increase healing, decrease aging, and assist in the rejuvenation of our joints, skin, brain, nervous system, pancreas, liver, and hair.

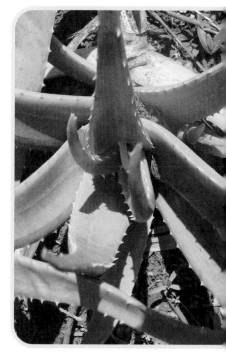

Glutathione

Aloe vera is potent in activating the liver to produce more glutathione. Glutathione is an antioxidant that is critical to the production of white blood cells. Typically, high amounts of glutathione in the body, along with a high dietary intake of vitamins B6, B9, and B12, will tend to lower dangerous homocysteine levels. Elevated homocysteine levels are a byproduct of an underlying nanobacteria infection and have been associated with nearly a hundred medical conditions.

Keeping the Kidneys Healthy

Aloe vera is a tonic adaptogen—adaptogens keep our vital organs healthy. They help balance blood sugar and enhance the liver, digestive system, and skin.

Supplementing the diet with aloe, aloe extracts (500+ mg daily), and arabinogalactan (polysaccharide gum sugar) supplements (500+ mg daily) has been shown to help decrease the need for kidney dialysis, as mentioned in Emil Mondoa's and Mindy Kitei's book *Sugars That Heal.*

Topical Applications: Healing the Skin

Aloe has been used topically to treat the following:

Abrasions

Acne

Arthritis—joint relief may be experienced by simple topical application

Athlete's foot

Blemishes

Brown spots

Burns

Eczema

Hemorrhoids

Insect bites

Insect stings

Jellyfish stings

Poison ivy

Poison oak

Psoriasis

Rashes

Scarring

Skin allergies

Skin cancer

Skin infections

Staph infections

Stretch marks

Stinging nettle

Sunburn

Varicose veins

Wounds

In my experience, the key in treating the skin topically with aloe vera appears to be keeping the aloe gel on the area for several hours each day, as opposed to just rubbing the gel on or using a lotion.

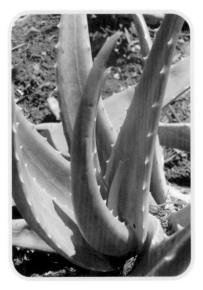

In both animals and humans, aloe vera's ability to heal and even prevent skin damage has been extensively researched and proven. Slabs of fresh aloe vera gel can be applied and left directly on sunburns, skin cancer, eczema, and psoriasis for several hours with positive effects.

Langerhans white blood cells coordinate the healing of damaged skin. In severe skin damage, the Langerhans cells may be suppressed. When applied topically, aloe vera also stimulates the production of Langerhans cells both locally and systemically.

What to Look For . . .

Aloe Vera Product Types

Aloe vera leaves are usually a foot or two in length and dull-green in color. They have a succulent texture and are rich with gel inside. Aloe gel can taste bitter or it can have hardly any taste at all.

When purchasing aloe vera look the following characteristics:

1. Purchase organic aloe vera.

2. Select fresh aloe vera leaves in preference to bottled aloe vera. Only fresh aloe vera maintains the strong antifungal components that aloe contains. Bottled aloe vera should at least be enzymatically "stabilized." Typically, the healing polysaccharide we know as mannose in aloe vera is destroyed by processing.

3. Select aloe leaves that are thick with gel and free of white speckles. Generally, the aloe variety with no white speckles in the leaf is superior to the ones with them.

Below is a list of aloe vera products to look for on the Internet or in your health food store or supplement shop.

Whole aloe vera leaves: Fresh aloe vera gel is superior to all other forms of aloe. It is more potent; its antifungal enzymes are still intact, and it has better flavor.

Bottled aloe vera gel

Dried aloe vera powder: A great product to fight chronic bladder infections. Take 750–1,500 milligrams per day

Acemannan (mannose extract)

Aloe vera alcohol tinctures

Aloe vera lotions (some exceptional formulas also contain MSM)

How to Use Aloe Vera

The gel of raw, fresh aloe vera has a mild, slightly bitter flavor due to the presence of high concentrations of polysaccharides.

Aloe vera is best when filleted. Cut the portion you desire to eat from the aloe leaf, remove the thorns on either side, and separate the gel from the skin with your knife.

Once the gel is removed from the inner leaf, it may be combined with other foods in smoothies, elixirs, salads, or other food preparations. Aloe vera combines well with high-antioxidant foods and superfoods like bee pollen, goji berries, fresh noni, and raw chocolate in all types of recipes, and it has a synergistic effect with whole-food, antioxidant-rich, green superfood formulas such as Pure Synergy®. Try mixing tiny cubes of raw aloe vera gel into a salsa, or blend up pieces of the raw gel into soups, spreads, and dips (yes, the gel can be cubed). Add the benefits of this traditional healing food to any raw dish you can imagine!

Once the gel has been removed and filleted from the outer leaf, the thin gel remaining on the inner surface of the leaf may be applied to the skin as a moisturizing lotion, suntan lotion, or as a soothing relief from minor burns.

Aloe vera leaves keep best when left in a bowl in indirect light at room temperature (not in the refrigerator).

Warning: Due to its strong effects in cleansing the liver, pregnant women and young children should not take aloe vera internally.

Topical Applications

Aloe vera has tremendous topical applications for burns and chronic skin challenges. The key to using aloe vera effectively is exposing the gel by removing the skin and then placing the gel on the affected area for several hours without removing it. Simply rubbing aloe briefly on an area will not be effective.

Athlete's Foot and Foot Fungus

Most forms of foot fungus can be overcome by removing the aloe skin and blending the fresh inner gel with spring water into a slurry, then pouring the slurry into a bucket and soaking one's feet in the bucket for several hours a day for six weeks.

If you have fungus under the nails of your hands or feet, this aloe gel soaking should be done daily along with a topical application (when the affected area is clean and dry) of neem alcohol extract, pau d'arco alcohol extract, and 70 percent DMSO (dimethyl sulfoxide) sprayed on top of that. The area should be left to dry for fifteen to twenty minutes before socks or clothing touch the area. DMSO is a chemical solvent and should not be used haphazardly. Be sure to read Dr. Morton Walker's book *DMSO: Nature's Healer* before using DMSO.

Growing Aloe Vera

My experience growing aloe vera is fairly extensive. I have grown aloe in poor soil, clay-like soil, potting soil, 50 percent beach sand, desert sand, and in rich tropical soil. Aloe seems to prefer beach sand mixed 50-50 with some potting soil and enough alkaline minerals (such as calcium) to keep the soil somewhat alkaline. I have consistently found the best results with this combination. Aloe likes to be in well-drained soil and get reasonable soaks of water every now and again. I always let my aloes' soils almost dry out in between watering or rain. It is much easier to overwater than underwater this special plant.

If you live in a tropical or subtropical zone, grow your aloe outdoors in indirect sunlight. Plant them in places that require little care or maintenance. Aloes grow themselves and require little attention. In colder climates, keep your potted aloes near the window during the cold months and outside in indirect sunlight during the warmer months.

Harvesting leaves from your plant does not harm it as long as at least three strong leaves remain. Remove the leaves lowest to the ground first. Attempt to peel the leaf off the stalk. Most of the time you will be able to peel it off without damaging the leaf or the stalk at all. If you are unable to do this, simply use a knife and cut the aloe leaf near the stalk.

I have used Dead Sea salt and Dead Sea salt extracts as fertilizer for my aloe plants. I usually add a pinch of Dead Sea salt per gallon of water and water my aloe with this four to six times a year. Once a year, I pour the Dead Sea salt extract into a freshly dug hole next to my aloe patch. I cover this hole back up with fresh dirt after I pour the extract in.

Dead Sea salt extracts may be made by adding a 10 percent solution of sodium hydroxide by the drop to a one-gallon (4-liter) water-based solution containing 1–2 heaping tablespoons of Dead Sea salt. Add sodium hydroxide by the drop until the pH of the gallon hits 10–10.5 and then decant (keeping the precipitate intact) with distilled water to bring the pH back down. I have then used this precipitate and the distilled water, when the pH hits 7, as fertilizer for the aloe.

Aloe Vera Recipes

To Prepare (Fillet) Aloe Vera

Starting from the thickest part (base) to the thinnest (top), choose the amount of aloe you want to use. Cut off a chunk, cut the sharp edges off the sides, then fillet the skin off the top and bottom. Use the slimy, clear parts for your recipes. This is the precious aloe gel.

Avo's Lemonade

To a 3/4 full (1¹/2 liters) blender filled with spring water, add:

    1/2 prepared aloe leaf (remove skin, keep the gel)

    1 whole lemon, with the outer rind removed (keep the white pith)

    1 whole lime, with the outer rind removed (keep the white pith)

    5 pinches sea salt

    3–5 droppersful of David Wolfe's wild goji berry extract
       (or 3–5 pinches of goji berry powder)

    2 tbsp. agave syrup

Blend and strain. Serve on ice.

Strawberry Orange Aloe Drink

Put prepared aloe gel in a blender.

> Add fresh squeezed orange juice until the blender is 3/4 full
>
> Add 1 cup organic strawberries
>
> Add 1/2 cup goji berries

Mix with water if desired. Blend, strain, and serve cold.

Hydrating Aloe Delight

> Juice 1 cucumber in a juicer
>
> Juice 1–2 apples in a juicer
>
> Juice of 1 freshly squeezed lemon
>
> 2–3 pinches Himalayan salt

Blend all these ingredients with prepared aloe gel in a blender.

Add water and ice if desired.

Supergreen Power Aloe Smoothie

> Add your favorite green powder (select your favorite brand containing superfoods, superherbs, vegetables, grasses, seaweeds, etc.)
>
> freshly squeezed organic orange juice
>
> 2 organic kale leaves or favorite leafy green vegetable
>
> prepared aloe gel

Blend well in a high-speed blender. Add water if desired.

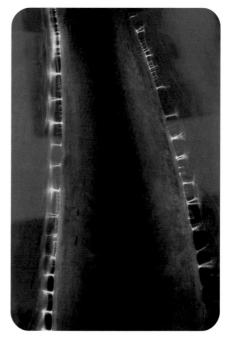

Twinkling Pink Aloe Cleanser

2–3 tbsp. flax oil

1 whole grapefruit (peeled)

inside gel from 1/2 an aloe vera leaf (not skin)

1/2 cup spring water (or just enough to blend)

2 tbsp. sweetener of choice (NoniLand™ honey, Manuka honey, agave syrup, or a few drops of stevia—sweeten to taste)

Blend all ingredients together in high-speed blender, pour into glass, chill if desired, and serve!

Chocolate–Vanilla Bean Dream Recipe

4 cups of your favorite liquid—we recommend water, hot or cold tea, fresh coconut water, or any nut milk

3 tbsp. raw cacao powder

1 tbsp. maca or Maca Extreme if you dare!

1 tsp. cinnamon

1 tbsp. raw cacao nibs

2 tbsp. coconut butter

1 tbsp. wild jungle peanuts

1–2 tbsp. sweetener (we suggest yacon syrup, amber or dark agave, and/or raw honey)

1 tbsp. hempseed

1 small pinch Celtic sea salt

1/2 tsp. ginger (optional)

1/2–1 tsp. cayenne pepper (optional)

1/4–1/2 leaf fresh aloe vera gel

1/2 fresh vanilla bean

    3–5 capsules (1500 mg) reishi mycelium (reishi mushroom powder), open capsules and pour powder in (optional, for immune energy boost!)

    1–3 cups organic frozen berries depending on how thick you like your smoothie

Mix all ingredients in a blender and serve. Serves 4.

Oh WOW Cacao—Superfood Greens Booster!

    4 cups liquid (we recommend water, hot or cold tea, fresh coconut water, or any nut milk—hemp, almond, etc.)

    3 tbsp. raw cacao powder

    1 tbsp. raw maca, red maca, or Maca Extreme if you dare!

    1 tbsp. raw cacao nibs

    2 tbsp. coconut butter

    1 tbsp. wild jungle peanut butter

    2 tbsp. green powdered superfoods (select your favorite brand containing superfoods, superherbs, vegetables, grasses, seaweeds, etc.)

    1–2 tbsp. sweetener (we suggest yacon syrup, amber or dark agave, and/or raw honey (depending on how sweet you like your smoothies)

    1 tbsp. hempseed

    1 small pinch Celtic sea salt

    1/4–1/2 leaf fresh aloe vera gel

    1/2 tbsp. spirulina

    1–3 cups organic frozen fruit (depending on how thick you prefer your smoothie)

Blend all ingredients in a blender. Serves 2–4.

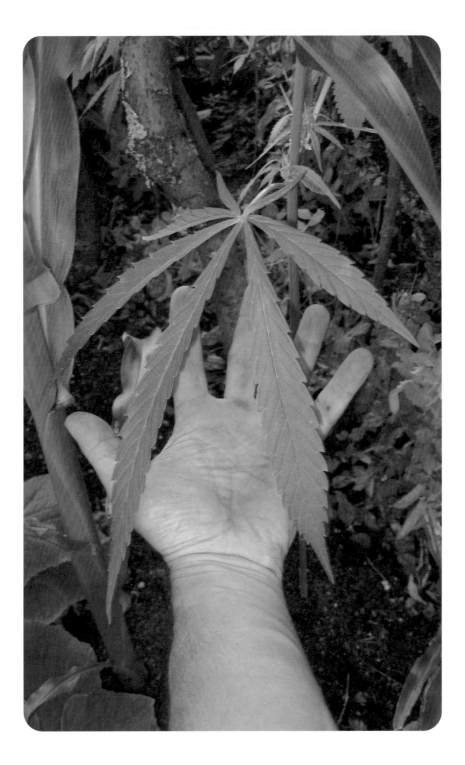

Hempseed
Superfood of the Future

Latin Names:

Major Varieties: *Cannabis sativa* L.,
        Cannabis indica

Common Names:

Hempseed, hempnut

Superfood Type:

Seed

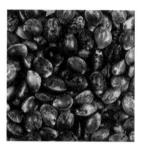

History, Facts, and Legends

Hemp belongs to the same family of plants as mulberry (otherwise known as *Moraceae*). The mulberry family is known for its genetic and chromosomal complexity, which is likely what allows this family of plants to survive in nearly every climate on Earth.

Hemp is a tough plant believed to originate in Central Asia. It can be grown in practically any ecosystem in the world. Although usually three to six feet in height at full growth, hemp can reach a height of over fifteen feet! Hemp does not require any of the pesticides or herbicides that are used to keep weak plants alive. Only eight out of nearly a hundred known common crop pests may cause problems, and these can be dealt with by natural means. Hemp also naturally suppresses weeds due to its fast growth and the development of a canopy. And on top of all of this, the hemp plant produces a superfood as a seed.

Hemp and Civilization

Without [hemp rope] how could water be drawn from the well? What would scribes, copyists, secretaries, and writers do without it [hemp paper]? Would not official documents and rent-rolls disappear? Would not the noble art of printing perish?

—François Rabelais (1495–1553), French humanist and satirist during the Renaissance; quoted in *At the Edge of History* by William Irwin Thompson

Hemp production is probably the oldest industry on the planet, going back more than ten thousand years. The *Columbia History of the World* states that the oldest relic of human industry is a piece of hemp fabric dating back to approximately 8000 BC. The oldest Chinese agricultural treatise, the *Xia Xiao Zheng*, written in the sixteenth century BC, discusses hemp as one of the primary crops grown in ancient China. Since the beginning of human history, the cultivation and use of hemp has also occurred in the native cultures of North America and Europe and in the great civilizations of India, Sumeria, Mesopotamia, Persia, Egypt, and Central America.

Hemp falls into the *Cannabis* genus. The Persians called hemp *kanab,* and the Greeks *kanabis* (from which we derive not only the English word "cannabis" but also the word "canvas"). The Germans call it *hanf* or *hampf;* the Dutch *hennep;* the Danish *hamp;* the Swedes *hampa;* and the Chinese *huo ma ren.*

Hemp has played a vital role in agriculture and culture—especially in America. The "hamp" place name (New Hampshire, Hampstead, Hampton, etc.) references locations where hemp was once grown.

George Washington and Thomas Jefferson both grew hemp on their farms and Ben Franklin owned a hemp paper mill. Hemp continued as a massive agricultural crop in North America until the late 1930s. Hempseed is literally as American as apple pie.

The Hemp Conspiracy

In 1937 *Popular Science* magazine called hemp "The New Billion-Dollar Crop." A machine that simplified the hemp papermaking process had just been invented. But the promise of hemp was never fulfilled.

In the early 1930s one of the great media conspiracies of the twentieth century unfolded. Newspaper publisher William Randolph Hearst, along with DuPont Corporation, a group of petroleum interests, the American cotton-growing lobby, international bankers, and a group of ignorant politicians, led a crusade to ban hemp.

The Hearst family had acquired millions of acres of forestland that it intended to turn into paper for publishing and Pierre DuPont held patent rights to the sulfuric-acid, wood-pulp paper process. Also, in 1937 DuPont patented nylon rope (to replace hemp rope) made from synthetic petrochemicals. The petroleum industry did not want any competition from hemp rope, nor did they want to compete against inexpensive hempseed biodiesel fuel, so Hearst used his power as a publisher to sway public opinion about hemp and marijuana.

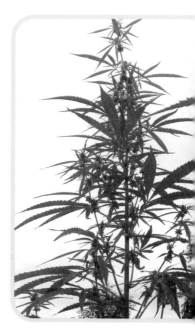

With the help of U.S. Treasury Secretary Andrew Mellon the United States Congress passed the Marijuana Tax Act in 1937, which placed a prohibitive, elaborate set of rules around the growing, handling, and distributing of hemp. This was possible because marijuana is a subspecies of hemp known for its elevated psychoactive and medicinal THC content. A violation of any of the 1937 Tax Act rules would result in a penalty of up to $2,000 (in 1937 currency) or up to five years in prison. This legislation essentially ground the hemp production industry to a halt in America.

Hemp was briefly legalized again during World War II. The United States government produced the film *Hemp for Victory* to encourage farmers to grow the crop. Nearly a million acres of hemp were grown in the Midwest to support the war effort. But hemp farming was shut down after the war. Then, due to pressure brought by the same special interests as before, came the *Comprehensive Drug Abuse Prevention and Control Act of 1970* that outlawed marijuana altogether and made little distinction between hemp and marijuana.

Hemp or Marijuana?

Hemp and marijuana are both classified as *Cannabis sativa,* a species with hundreds of subspecies varieties.

That the hemp plant, *Cannabis sativa,* may be used as a superfood initially surprises some people. The government and media have largely restricted knowledge of hemp to its unique variants of marijuana. Marijuana, with its leaf and flower content of the psychoactive substance delta-9-tetrahydrocannabinol (THC), has become illegal in most of the Western world and labeled a "drug," while other very serious and extremely dangerous drugs such as hard liquor and pharmaceuticals (with known dangerous side effects) are legal.

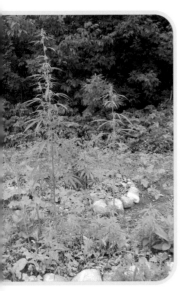

Industrial hemp is bred to maximize fiber, seed, and/or oil, while marijuana varieties seek to maximize THC. Hemp has a typical THC level of between 0.05 and 1 percent in its flowers. Marijuana has a THC level that ranges from 3 to 20 percent in its flowers. Because of the low THC content of hemp flowers, it would take over a dozen joints smoked in a dozen minutes to feel even a slight effect.

We are often told that hemp looks so similar to marijuana that hemp growers could hide marijuana plants in their fields. The truth is that hemp's low levels of THC immediately ruin marijuana's THC levels and female bud production. If hemp does pollinate any nearby marijuana, the result will always be lower THC marijuana. Marijuana cultivated outdoors must be grown far away from hemp to avoid producing poor quality, seedy flowers (buds) and to prevent cross-pollination.

The Many Facets of the Superplant Hemp

All parts of the hemp plant are useful. Hemp can be used to make virtually anything that is currently made of cotton, timber, or petroleum. Hemp can be used to produce nearly every major category of commercial product. And hemp produces a superfood seed. Consider the various aspects of the hemp plant that can be used in the following ways:

Hempseed and Hemp Leaves

The hempseed is a complete protein source. The oil from hempseed has the highest percentage of essential fatty acids of nearly any seed on Earth. Hempseed typically contains over twenty trace minerals. It naturally sprouts on the hemp plant late in the growing season (during the autumn), lowering phytic acid and increasing enzymes, which make the seed even more digestible. Hempseed's essential fatty acid and protein profile provides a healthy alternative to fish, which is becoming increasingly risky to eat, given rising mercury and PCB contamination.

Hemp leaves are also edible. They contain a high percentage of silica, which is useful in building strong bones and beautiful skin, hair, and nails. Hemp leaf is rich in fiber. One side of the hemp leaf is soft and the other side is abrasive, so as the leaf is eaten and the fiber moves through the body, the sides of the leaf churn through the digestive tract, scrubbing and softly cleaning the intestines.

Dried hemp leaf tea has phenomenal taste as well as antimicrobial action. In my experiments with making tea and leaving different teas exposed to the atmosphere in my home for over a week, I've found that hemp leaf tea keeps microbes from growing in it even better than the most powerful herbs available, including powerful antimicrobial Amazonian herbs such as pau d'arco and cat's claw.

Hemp Body Care

Thanks to its nourishing oil, hemp is booming in the personal hygiene industry with hemp found in soaps, shampoos, lotions, lip balms, bath oils, personal lubricants, and more. Companies such as Dr. Bronner's have fought long and hard against hemp persecution in order to keep hemp body-care products on store shelves for all of us.

Hemp Textiles (Clothing and Fabrics)

The hemp plant is made up of the planet's strongest natural fibers. Hemp was the first crop ever cultivated for textile production. One acre of hemp will produce more textiles than two acres of cotton. In addition, hemp is four times warmer than cotton, four times more water-absorbent, and has three times the tensile strength of cotton.

Hemp is also a far safer crop to grow than cotton. Cotton is typically sprayed with chemical pesticides seven times each growing season, causing all sorts of environmentally disastrous problems including the contamination of groundwater and ill health in humans, nearby plants, animals, and insects. In the United States, cotton occupies 1 percent of the farmland but uses 50 percent of all pesticides. As much as 38 percent of the pesticides found in cotton clothing can be absorbed when one perspires in it.

Hemp textiles are stronger, more durable, more insulated, more mildew- and mold-resistant, and easier to produce than textiles made out of cotton. Hemp clothing breathes well, moving moisture away from the body better than cotton. Clothing that consists of at least one-half hemp fibers provides protection from overexposure to the sun's UV rays.

Hemp Paper

China was the world's first paper maker. The ancient Chinese used hemp to make paper nearly two thousand years ago. Until 1883, more than 75 percent of the world's paper was made with hemp fiber.

Hemp can yield three to eight dry tons of fiber per acre, four times more than what an average forest yields. Hemp can replace wood fiber, saving our forests from destruction. Most trees take nearly twenty years to mature—hemp takes four months. Paper made from hemp lasts for centuries, compared to twenty-five to eighty years for paper made from wood pulp. Hemp planting not only reduces deforestation, it improves the soil upon which it is grown. By producing hemp, we can save the forests that provide our fresh water, wildlife habitats, recreation opportunities, oxygen, carbon traps (reducing atmospheric damage), and natural beauty.

Hemp's low lignin content reduces the need for acids used in pulping, and its creamy color lends itself to environmentally friendly bleaching with hydrogen peroxide instead of harsh, environmentally dangerous chlorine-bleaching chemicals.

Hemp fiber paper resists decomposition better than any natural material. Hemp paper can be recycled ten times, while wood-based paper can only be recycled twice. Hemp paper more than fifteen hundred years old has been found.

Hemp Rope

Hemp rope has been used to make cloth and rope for over ten thousand years. Hemp ropes are known for their strength and durability. The production and use of hemp rope is one of the basic technologies that made sailing possible. Imagine sailing without any rope or string! Hemp rope is produced from hemp fibers.

Hemp Plastics

Eco-friendly hemp can replace nearly all the toxic petrochemical products. Hempseed can be used to manufacture biodegradable plastic products, cellophane, recycled plastic mixed with hemp for injection-molded products, resins, oil paints, varnishes, inks, solvents, lubricants, putty, and coatings, to name a few examples. Over two million cars currently in use in this country have hemp composite parts for doors, dashboards, roof racks, and other parts produced from hemp grown outside of the United States.

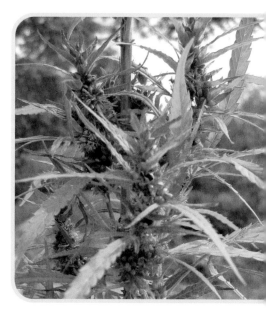

Hemp Building Materials

The core of the hemp stalk is used to produce fiberboard, insulation, carpet, fiberglass substitutes, cement blocks, concrete, stucco, and mortar. The hemp building materials MDF (medium density fiber) composite boards, tested by Washington State University Wood Materials and Engineering Laboratory, proved to be two and a half times stronger than wood MDF composites. Hemp composite boards were also three times more elastic than wood composite boards. Elasticity is the factor that determines whether or not a nail can be driven into the board. Another advantage is that water does not penetrate MDF hemp boards.

Hemp Fuel

The original diesel engine was designed to run on plant oils such as hempseed oil. Any diesel engine can still run on hemp oil or refined biodiesel made from hemp oil.

Hemp is the perfect source for ethanol gasoline fuel as well. It produces more biomass than any other plant—ten tons per acre in approximately four months. According to the U.S. Department of Energy, hemp as a biomass fuel producer requires the least specialized growing and processing procedures of all hemp products. The development of biofuels can actually eliminate our consumption of fossil fuels and nuclear power.

When hemp is burned as fuel, any carbon dioxide released from the burning hemp matches the carbon dioxide the plant had beneficially taken from the environment during its lifetime, creating a closed carbon cycle that slows down the effects of atmospheric pollution.

Hemp Vehicles

In 1941 Henry Ford produced an experimental automobile with a hemp-resin body composed of 70 percent cellulose fibers from hemp. The auto was lighter than typical metal vehicle framing, giving it greater fuel efficiency. The car body could absorb blows ten times as great as steel without denting. The car was designed to run on hemp-ethanol fuel. Because of the petroleum-backed smear campaigns and the ban on both hemp and alcohol, the car was never mass-produced.

Saving the Planet with Hemp

Because of its multiplicity of uses, the hemp plant is legendary among ecologically oriented individuals and entrepreneurs involved in environmentally friendly businesses. The Union of Concerned Scientists has stated that 80 percent of our ongoing ecological problems are caused by four human activities:

1. Driving cars and light trucks;
2. Meat and poultry production;
3. Nonorganic agriculture; and
4. Home construction and maintenance.

By incorporating hemp into the design and manufacturing process, the ecological harm in each of these categories is reduced or eliminated. All products made solely from hemp fibers are biodegradable, compostable, and recyclable.

Benefits

Leading researchers and medical doctors consider hemp to be one of the most nutritious food sources on the planet. The hardiness and nutritional power of hempseed could significantly address the planet's protein needs and starvation problems.

As exposure levels to artificial chemicals, pesticides, and radioactive materials increase, more and more people are becoming interested in eating low on the food chain (as opposed to eating animal products such as meat, large ocean fish, crustaceans, and dairy that are high on the food chain where toxins accumulate)—this means eating more and more plants.

The side effects of eating animal products, such as excessive cholesterol, saturated fat, and weight gain, along with increasingly poor quality and taste as well as artificial chemical use (pesticides, injected hormones, animal vaccinations, etc.) are becoming an overwhelming problem, causing millions of people to seek more humane, sustainable alternatives with vegetarian, vegan, and raw-food sources of protein and fat. One of the best sources of plant protein and fat is found in hempseed.

In terms of its average nutrient content, shelled hempseed is 35 percent protein, 47 percent fat, and 12 percent carbohydrate.

Hempseeds contain all the essential amino acids and essential fatty acids necessary to maintain healthy human life. No other single plant source has the essential amino acids in such an easily digestible form, or has the essential fatty acids in as perfect a ratio to meet human nutritional needs.

Packed with 33 to 37 percent pure digestible protein, raw hempseed, with all their original life-force energy and enzymes intact, are one of nature's richest sources of complete protein. Only algae such as spirulina, AFA blue-green algae, and marine phytoplankton exceed hemp in protein.

Approximately 47 percent of each hempseed is comprised of "good fats," with an ideal balance of omega-3 (alpha-linolenic acid) and omega-6 essential fatty acids (linoleic acid and gamma-linolenic acid).

The carbohydrate content of shelled hempseed is 11.5 percent and its sugar content is 2 percent. Of the shelled hempseed carbohydrate, 6 percent is in the form of fiber. The fiber content of hempseed flour is the highest of all commercially grown seeds. In addition to containing the basic human nutrient groups, hempseed have a high content of vitamin E (three times higher than flax) in the form of alpha-, beta-, gamma-, and delta-tocopherol and alpha-tocotrienols.

Hempseed are also an outstanding source of monounsaturated omega-9 fatty acids, which are considered a healthy energy source and a quality beautifying oil.

Hempseed is a good source of brain building, liver-supporting lecithin. Lecithin is a lipid substance (fat-oil) composed primarily of choline and inositol. It is found in all living cells as a major component of cell membranes. The term "lecithin" is derived from the Greek word *lekithos* meaning "egg," as lecithin was first discovered in eggs.

Hempseed is one of the few seeds that contains chlorophyll. Present inside each hempseed are infant green leaves that will eventually open and grow as the seed sprouts.

The THC found in various concentrations in the hemp genus is medicinally useful to individuals with chronic pain and nausea such as cancer patients.

Protein

Amino acids are chemical units of "building blocks" that make up protein. Next to water, protein makes up the greatest portion of the body's weight. Protein builds muscles, ligaments, tendons, organs, glands, nails, hair, body fluids, and nearly all aspects of microscopic cellular machinery. Protein is essential to the growth of bones.

Proteins themselves can act as neurotransmitters or precursors to neurotransmitters enabling all of our cells to receive and transmit messages.

Protein is useful not just for building muscle and strength, but also for endurance, balanced blood sugar and brain chemistry, neurological health, rapid healing, building strong bones, detoxification, and nearly every other aspect of healthy living.

The challenge we face is that "high-protein" animal foods are becoming more and more difficult to obtain. High-protein "wild game" is increasingly rare, and factory farmed beef, chicken, and fish are lower in protein and higher in fat and toxins. Factory animal farming is environmentally, emotionally, and psychologically dysfunctional, the impact of which is making us all aware that we must move away from toxic sources of protein.

Hempseed, unlike commonly available animal protein, is a pure, raw source of complete protein. It never needs to be cooked to kill bacteria, so all of its vital components remain intact.

Hempseed protein can also be more readily absorbed than animal protein because it blends easily into water, beverages, smoothies, shakes, and salad dressings without coagulation or heat. Hempseed is easy on the digestive system.

Of the protein fraction of the total hempseed, 65+ percent consists of globular edestin—the highest concentration found in the plant kingdom. The word "edestin" comes from the Greek word *edestos,* which means edible. Edestin is considered by many scientists and researchers to be the most edible and easily digestible form of protein in the food chain.

The other 35 percent of the protein in hemp is albumin, which is also considered one of the more easily digested forms of protein.

Edestin and albumin are "soft" broad-spectrum proteins that are hypoallergenic (low in allergy-forming reactions within the population). Many people are allergic to common high-protein foods such as whey and soy.

Edestin and the Immune System

Edestin is a plant globulin. Globulins are simple globular proteins constructed entirely from amino acids. Nearly all antibodies, enzymes, hormones, hemoglobin molecules, and fibrogin (which converts to the blood-clotting agent fibrin) are globular proteins and can be constructed out of edestin.

Globulins are divided into three classes: alpha, beta, and gamma globulins. Alpha and beta globulins are super-transporters that carry protein and information from one part of the body to another via the blood.

They cart the raw materials required to build new tissues as well as replace injured tissues.

Gamma globulins work on the immune system and are divided into five classes of antibodies called immunoglobulins. All are formed to combat specific cell-invading microbes. These globulins are responsible for both the natural and acquired immunity a person has against foreign microbes. They are essential to a healthy immune system.

Gamma globulins comprise the first line of defense against infection. They are antibodies programmed by white blood cells and replicated by white blood cell clones known as plasma cells. These gamma globulin antibodies destroy antigens (microbes) such as nanobacteria, viruses, bacteria, toxic fungi, cancer cells, toxins, dead tissue, and internal waste debris. Antibodies are custom designed to neutralize or disintegrate only one specific type of antigen. These antibodies circulate in the lymph fluid and the blood (sometimes for years) awaiting near contact with the antigen they are made to destroy. Once they come within the vicinity of the antigen, the antibody initiates the release of a cascade of corrosive enzymes that pulverize the antigen surface.

One white blood cell can give birth to hundreds of clone plasma cells in just a few days. A mature plasma cell produces about two thousand antibodies every second during its few days of life. The body's ability to resist and recover from illness depends upon how rapidly it can produce massive amounts of antibodies to fend off an initial attack. This is how we develop and acquire immunity.

If the globulin protein-starting material is in short supply, nutrient transport is impaired and the army of antibodies may be too small to prevent the symptoms of sickness from setting in.

Because hempseed is the world's best source of globulin-building materials (edestin), eating hempseed will ensure the body has the reservoir of globulin resources necessary to transport raw materials and support the immune system and immune response.

Essential Fatty Acids

Essential fatty acids (EFAs) are considered "essential" because our body does not manufacture them independently, nor can they be created from other fats or oils in our diet. The presence of essential fatty acids in our diet is now considered a critical aspect of maintaining great health for a lifetime.

Essential fatty acids are powerful antioxidants that protect our skin from excessive sun exposure. They also play an important role in improving our immune system due to their potential anti-inflammatory properties. They help us burn excess fat by delivering readily available energy that helps carry and remove toxins from the skin, intestinal tract, kidneys, and lungs. EFAs nourish and feed the brain and eyes, which are made up of a large fraction of omega-3 fatty acids. EFAs also lubricate our cardiovascular system, reducing the threat of heart disease and stroke.

Hemp is one of very few plants that contains significant amounts of the following essential fatty acids: omega-6 (linoleic acid and GLA) as well as omega-3 (ALA). The oil fraction of the overall hempseed normally contains about 80 percent of these essential polyunsaturated fatty acids, with omega-6 and 3 in the ideal ratios of approximately 3:1 or 4:1. The perfect ratio of omega-6 to omega-3 is 3.38:1, closely approximating the 3:1 ratio recommended for the human diet by America's leading dietary fat and oil expert Udo Erasmus and the 4:1 average ratio recommended by the World Health Organization (WHO), Sweden, and Japan. Hempseed are the only food known that contain these ideal ratios. Fish oil and flaxseed oil are rich in omega-3, but not omega-6. Almost all the commonly consumed nuts and seeds are rich in omega-6, but not omega-3.

The omega-3 content of hempseed increases when the plant is grown in the extreme northern or southern hemispheres. The cooler the climate, the higher the need for polyunsaturated fatty acids, especially omega-3s, which are well-represented not only in hempseed but also in cold-water fish, marine phytoplankton, krill, flaxseeds, walnuts, noni seeds, sacha inchi, blue-green algae, and many other interesting sources. Omega-3 fatty acids also protect us from overexposure to the sun, which is particularly strong in the extreme northern and southern hemispheres in the summer.

Scientific research has found that coconut oil appears to increase the effectiveness of the omega-3 fatty acids in hempseed, so consuming hempseed with raw organic coconut oil is recommended.

Gamma-Linolenic Acid (GLA)

Hempseed, like spirulina, contains the super anti-inflammatory, essential fatty acid known as gamma-linolenic acid (GLA).

GLA has been shown to inhibit the formation of inflammatory prostaglandins (short-lived hormones) and fatty arachidonate metabolites of digestion.

GLA is also known to help balance hormones. This means that hempseed may positively improve premenstrual syndrome (PMS) symptoms as well as mood swings. A deficiency of GLA has been shown to cause women to become oversensitive to their own prolactin hormone, causing breast pain.

Minerals

Hemp excels at absorbing minerals from the soil. Hempseed is an excellent source of major and trace minerals. Hempseed have been found to contain the following minerals*:

Phosphorous (an energy "battery" mineral, needed to improve bone density)

Potassium (an energy "action" mineral)

Magnesium (opens over 300 different detoxification pathways in the body)

Sulfur (primary beauty and longevity mineral)

Calcium (relaxes the digestive tract and muscular system, removes toxins)

Iron (a blood builder and oxygenator)

Manganese (a blood builder and oxygenator)

Zinc (a beauty mineral, supports the skin and liver)

Sodium (balances potassium, feeds the adrenals)

Silicon (a beauty mineral, needed to improve bone density)

Copper (part of the vitamin C complex, reverses gray hair)

Platinum (an enzymatic master mineral)

---

*This mineral list is derived from *Drugs Masquerading as Foods* by Suzar. The parenthetical comments have been added by David Wolfe.

> Boron (assists with calcium assimilation, normalizes hormones during menopause)
> Nickel (plays a key role in enzyme metabolism)
> Germanium (an antiviral, immune-supporting mineral)
> Tin (helps reverse male pattern baldness)
> Iodine (a thyroid mineral, reverses hypothyroidism)
> Chromium (a pancreatic mineral)
> Silver (an antiviral, antifungal, antimicrobial mineral)
> Lithium (an alkaline, mood-improving mineral)

Sulfur-Bearing Amino Acids

Hempseed protein delivers a balanced array of eighteen amino acids. An important aspect of hempseed protein is a high content of arginine (123 milligrams per gram of protein) and histidine (27 mg/g protein), both of which are important for growth during childhood, and of the sulfur-containing amino acids methionine (23 mg/g protein) and cysteine (16 mg/g protein), which are needed for proper enzyme formation.

Sulfur-bearing amino acids such as cysteine and methionine help the liver and nervous system detoxify poisons. They also improve the immune system, physical strength, flexibility, agility, complexion, hair luster, speed of healing, and the functionality of the liver and pancreas.

Delta-9-Tetrahydrocannabinol (THC)

Of all the kinds of hemp worldwide, only 2 to 3 percent is considered to be high enough in THC to be labeled "marijuana." Most of the THC and other psychoactive cannabinoids are found in the leaves and flowers.

Do Hempseed Contain THC?

In some cases hempseed do contain trace amounts of THC. Studies indicate that a dose as high as 5 milligrams of THC causes no psychoactive effects in an individual weighing 150 pounds. To ingest five milligrams of THC from hempseed containing two parts per million of THC, you would have to eat five pounds of hempseed in a day—an almost impossible feat that would still not cause a marijuana "high."

The United States government irrationally outlaws any hempseed products containing even trace amounts of THC. All hempseed delivered into the United States contains THC in amounts less than one part per million.

Generally, the strains of hemp plant selected for food use are those that produce little or no THC. These nutritional varieties of the hemp plant grow in temperate climates to heights of sixteen feet and, as with most agricultural grains, their seeds can be harvested in a conventional manner with a combine. Since modern handling and shelling of the seed minimize its contact with leaf resins, the shelled seed itself and the oil, nut butter, and other foods prepared from the seed are made with THC concentrations ranging from as low as one part per million to undetectable. These hemp products, when consumed in normally recommended amounts, should eliminate positive urine tests for THC. Studies conducted on older versions of hempseed oil found some to contain THC concentrations that resulted in positive urine tests.

What to Look For ...

Hempseed Product Types

To be imported into the United States of America, hempseed must be cracked out of their shells (hemp agriculture is illegal in most of the U.S. although the laws are shifting quickly as the general realized value of this plant continues to grow).

Imported hempseed and hemp protein products from Canada are currently available in the U.S. via the Internet, by mail order, and in some health food stores. Hemp food and body-care products currently available in the world market include:

Hempseed (shell removed)
Hempseed (whole)—Currently legal in many countries including the United Kingdom, but not legal in the United States as of this writing
Hempseed protein
Hempseed cold-pressed oil

Hempseed

Hempseed butter
Raw hempseed chocolate bars, protein, and energy bars
Raw hempseed ice cream
Hempseed salad dressings
Hempseed breads
Hempseed beer
Hempseed oil topical body-care products (soap, shampoo, etc.)

Of these hemp products, raw hemp protein powder is of particular importance for those requiring a high-protein diet. Made from raw hempseed (cold-pressed at less than 110 degrees), the remaining defatted hemp cake is then finely milled to contain protein powder, with much of the oil removed. Hemp protein is a balanced, "whole" protein, full of amino acids, vitamins, minerals, and antioxidants. Hemp's superior 66 percent edestin and 33 percent albumin protein structure is the highest in the plant kingdom.

How to Use Hempseed

Hempseed are great eaten alone as a snack. They go well sprinkled on salads. They blend well and add richness and flavor to smoothies and salad dressings.

Whole, unhulled hempseed may be soaked in water, if desired, to lower enzyme inhibitors typically found in seeds. They can then be deshelled and eaten or crushed into a milk, strained, and drunk fresh. I enjoy them both ways.

Hempseed can be easily added into superfood smoothies, fresh juices, raw chocolate (cacao) concoctions, and homemade salad dressings. Hempseed are richer in protein and more filling than most salad seeds such as sunflower and poppy seeds.

Recommended Dosages

- Beginner or child (ages 2–9): 15–30 grams a day
- Teen dose (ages 10–18): 30–50 grams a day
- Adult dose: 50–75 grams a day
- Super-Athlete dose: as much as 140 grams a day

Hempseed Recipes

Hemp Milk

1 cup hempseed

4 cups filtered water

1 pinch Celtic sea salt

1/4–1/2 vanilla bean

Blend all ingredients in blender and filter through a strainer, nut-milk bag, or other fine-mesh bag.

Add 1–3 tablespoons of a sweetener if you wish (raw honey, yacon root syrup, or agave nectar). Optional: add berries, peaches, and/or papaya.

If your hempseed are in the shell, soak them in water for 8 to 12 hours first, drain the water, wash the hempseed with more water, then blend and strain as directed above to remove the shells.

Add hemp milk to your smoothie or shake, your morning cereal, or to your coffee or tea. You can also drink hemp milk straight.

All Day Long Hemp Milk

1/2 cup hempseed

4 cups pure spring water

2 tbsp. milk thistle seeds, fine ground (a coffee grinder works well)

1 tbsp. spirulina

2 tbsp. agave nectar

1 raw vanilla bean (whole)

1 pinch Himalayan salt

This is another version of hemp milk with liver-supporting milk thistle seeds and spirulina. Blend until smooth, and strain through a strainer, nut-milk bag, or fine-mesh bag. Enjoy!

Hemp-Spirulina Snack

Add 1/2 cup spirulina and 1 teaspoon of Celtic sea salt to a 10-ounce bag of hempseed. Shake this mixture up and use as a salad topping; mix with olive oil or hemp oil and fresh lemon or apple cider vinegar for a delicious salad dressing; or eat it straight out of the bag with a spoon for a high-protein snack.

Hempseed Dressing

1/3 cup hempseed

1/4 hempseed oil

1/4 cup olive oil

3 tbsp. lemon juice

2 sprigs of parsley

2 tbsp. hempseed butter

2 tbsp. spirulina

2 tbsp. honey

Blend until smooth. I made this dressing on The Mad Mad House, a reality TV show I was on in 2005. It was a hit!

Cosmic Hempini Gravy

1/2 cup water

3 tbsp. lemon juice

2 tbsp. barley miso

1/3 cup hempseed

1 tsp. chopped ginger

2 tbsp. tahini

2 tbsp. olive oil

Blend until smooth. This recipe is the most nutritious gravy ever.

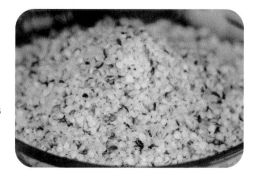

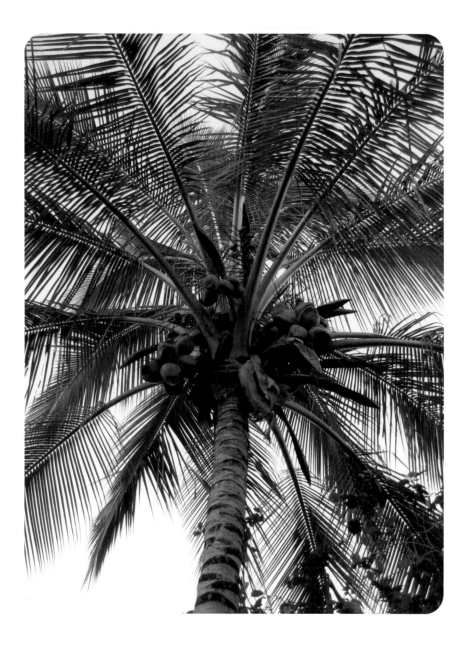

Coconuts
Symbol of Paradise

Latin Names:

Cocos nucifera

Common Names:

Coconut, Cocos, Coco

Superfood Type:

Seed

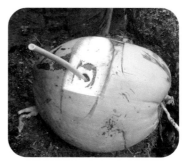

History, Facts, and Legends

> *Moreover, there were a great number of elephants in the island ... and the fruits having a hard rind, affording drinks. . . . All these things they received from the earth, and they employed themselves in constructing their temples, palaces, harbors, and docks.*

> —Plato, *Critias* (describing coconuts on the lost continent of Atlantis)

The coconut palm may grow to thirty meters in height, with giant pinnate leaves twelve to eighteen feet in length. As the old leaves die and/or break away from the palm, they do so cleanly, leaving a smooth coconut tree trunk. The term "coconut" refers to the giant seed of the coconut palm. An alternate spelling for coconut (seen in older books) is cocoanut—which is not to be confused with cocoa or cacao (chocolate)!

Coconut palms are prehistoric plants that are distantly related to grasses. Because they are a grass, coconut palms are extremely salt-tolerant and can grow right next to the ocean. Inland coconut palms can be directly fertilized with ocean water. Also like grasses, coconut palms can absorb nearly every mineral known to be useful in human nutrition.

Coconut palms thrive in sand and sandy soils, but can survive in clay soil conditions too. They love abundant sunlight, heavy rainfall (40–80 inches annually), and high humidity (60–80+ percent) for optimum growth. Coconuts have a difficult time in dry, arid conditions. Coconuts palm trees also need warmth, as they are intolerant to cold weather. They may grow but not fruit properly in areas of insufficient warmth and humidity like Southern California, where they make great houseplants.

Optimum warmth for coconut palm trees is between 70–90 degrees Fahrenheit. Coconut trees can survive winter temperatures in the range of 40–55 degrees and can even survive drops to freezing (32°F). Frost is usually fatal, although the trees have been known to recover from temperatures of 25 degrees.

Exactly where coconut palms originated is unknown, but a few scholars suggest it was the Philippines, which has the densest population of coconut palm trees of anywhere I have visited. The Philippines has the largest coconut production of any nation in the world.

The coconut is light and buoyant and can spread considerable distances by natural ocean currents. Coconuts can survive many months floating at sea. Coconuts still land on certain subtropical and temperate-climate beaches all over the world. It is not uncommon for a sproutable coconut to reach landfall on the beaches of Los Angeles even though this is outside the range of where coconuts will grow.

Coconuts were carried as a founder crop by ancient mariners throughout the world. Elaborate computer simulations of ocean currents and drift show that humans had to carry coconuts to America. Coconut palms grew on the southwest coast of Mexico when the Spanish arrived there, and were cultivated in all Mayan lands.

In the Hawaiian Islands, the coconut is regarded as a Polynesian introduction, first brought to the islands by early seafarers from their home islands in the South Pacific. Coconuts are now found all over the tropics between 26°N latitude and 26°S latitude.

Coconuts Can Save Your Life

In Sanskrit (the language of ancient India), the coconut palm is known as *kalpa vriksha*, meaning "the tree that supplies all that is needed to live."

Coconuts are one of the greatest gifts on this planet. No matter where you are, what you have done, how much you have mistreated your body, fresh young coconut flesh, coconut water, coconut cream, and/or coconut oil can save your life.

The coconut is a natural water filter that takes almost nine months to filter each liter (quart) of water in the shell. To get there, the water rises upward through innumerable fibers, which purify the water before it ends up in the sterile nut. This clear coconut water is one of the highest sources of electrolytes found in nature.

Young coconut water is nearly identical to human blood plasma, making it a universal donor. During the Pacific battles of World War II, between 1941 and 1945, both sides in the conflict used coconut water—siphoned directly from the coconut—to give emergency plasma transfusions to wounded soldiers. Plasma makes up 55 percent of human blood. The remaining 45 percent of our blood consists of hemoglobin—which is essentially transformed plant blood (chlorophyll). When we consume a drink consisting of 55 percent fresh coconut water and 45 percent fresh green-leaf juice (or wheatgrass juice, as Dr. Ann Wigmore recommended) we give ourselves an instant blood transfusion.

Coconuts are the most health enhancing in their young stage of growth. They contain a soft "spoon-meat," consisting mostly of a pure saturated fat that has the remarkable ability to rejuvenate age-related oxidative tissue damage, improve the functioning of the nervous system, increase breast-milk production, and restore male sexual fluids.

If you ever travel to a tropical country, you should drink and eat at least three or four young coconuts each day. In North America and Europe, young Thai coconuts are available in health food stores and in Asian

markets. These are "hybrid" nuts and are not as optimal as the wild tropical coconuts (such as those growing in Hawaii and Mexico) due to their
higher sugar-water content and lack of *prana* (vital life-force energy) in
the flesh. However, they are still quite useful and work especially well as
a base for smoothies or cultured beverages. Even organic young Thai
coconuts are now available.

Thai coconuts, like most imported coconuts, have been shaved down
from their original size and shape. In Asian markets, these plastic-wrapped
young white coconuts are easy to recognize because they are flat on one
side, cylindrical around the edges, and conical on top. When purchasing
these, seek out the newest coconuts that have come into the market. Any
mold or moisture underneath the plastic indicates that the nut is spoiled.

The brown, hairy coconuts most people are familiar with are mature
coconuts. They can contain a good quality of coconut water (not always),
yet the flesh is hard and fibrous, unlike the soft meat of the youthful stage.
The fibrous meat is less tasty and not as digestible, even though within
the fiber and protein is one of the most healing fat substances known.

Coconut Cream and Oil

The challenge with mature coconuts is that they contain a high quantity
of coarse protein and fiber (three times as much fiber as vegetables) that
surrounds the nourishing, cleansing coconut oil. This is solved by either
stone-grinding the fibrous copra (mature, hard, white coconut meat) into
a coconut cream, extracting the oil by heating the copra in water, and/or
by cold-pressing the healing fat out of the copra, thus concentrating its
essence into an oil. Truly raw coconut oil is produced when the coconut
copra is low-temperature dried, then cold-pressed. The oil is released in
the press and then bottled. Creamy white coconut oil becomes a clear oil
when it is warmed above 78 degrees Fahrenheit.

Coconut cream (sometimes called coconut butter) is derived from
mature coconuts containing hardened white flesh (copra). The copra is
shredded and collected. In a conching process with either stainless steel
or stone-grinders, the copra is micronized over a period of about twenty-
four hours, which breaks the copra down into a "cream cheese" type of
nut butter. (For clarity, there is no major difference between a fat and

an oil; the terms are used inter-changeably.)

Coconut oil and coconut cream have been used as food and medi-cine since the dawn of history. Ayurveda (the medicine of India) and the medicinal systems of Poly-nesia have long advocated the coconut's therapeutic and cosmetic properties. Coconut cream is so deli-cious that the biggest challenge is to try and stop eating it. By weight, coconut oil has fewer calories than any other fat source. Unlike the high-calorie, cholesterol-soaked,

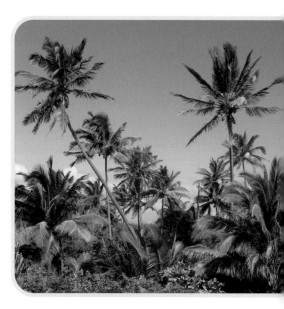

long-chain, saturated animal fats found in meat and dairy products, coconut cream and coconut oil are made of raw saturated fats containing mostly medium-chain fatty acids that the body can metabolize efficiently and convert to energy quickly.

Benefits

The following benefits may be derived from coconut products such as fresh young coconut flesh, coconut cream, and coconut oil:

- They improve digestion and absorption of fat-soluble vitamins and amino acids.
- They are valuable to the immune system as they contain healthy antivi-ral, antifungal, and antimicrobial saturated fatty acids, helping to nat-urally fight off viruses, bacteria, and fungal overgrowth.
- They improve the utilization of blood sugar and can lessen the symp-toms of hypoglycemia.
- They improve the absorption of the right kinds of calcium and magne-sium ions.
- They consist of 90+ percent raw saturated fat—a rare and important building block of every cell in the human body. Unlike long-chain

saturated animal fats (that have been associated with creating poor health), the saturated fat in coconut oil is in the form of medium-chain fatty acids (MCFAs). MCFAs support the immune system, the thyroid gland, the nervous system, the skin, and provide fast energy.

- They contain powerful antioxidants in the form of raw saturated fats and oils. Coconut oil contains the most lauric acid (a powerful antiviral substance) of any plant source.
- They help the body use the essential fatty acids (omega-3, omega-6) and other fatty acids and phospholipids (e.g. choline, lecithin, etc.) more efficiently. You can and should take coconut oil at the same time as omega-3 fatty acids or superfoods rich in omega-3 fatty acids such as hempseed, marine phytoplankton powder, AFA algae, etc. Coconut oil and omega-3 fatty acids are twice as effective when taken together as when taken alone.
- They help regulate and support healthy hormone production.
- They are a nutritional precursor to the anti-aging hormone compound known as pregnenolone.
- They increase the speed of the thyroid, thus allowing the body to drop excess weight and accumulated toxins. Contrary to some previously held beliefs, coconut cannot be stored in the body as fat; it actually needs to be burned up on the spot, which helps fire up our excess fat-burning metabolism immediately.
- They help displace toxic hydrogenated trans-fatty acids (e.g., partially hydrogenated soybean oil).
- They restore natural saturated fat levels to the skin, subcutaneous fat layers, and to the individual cell membranes. The saturated fats in coconut products are also vital for the health of growing nervous systems in children.
- They increase metabolism and help with weight loss due to the presence of medium-chain saturated fatty acids present in coconut products. Farm animals fed coconuts and coconut oil are never obese. When fed partially hydrogenated soybean oil and other rancid fats, the animals gain weight.
- They contain no appreciable levels of cholesterol and actually support cardiovascular health. This is based on research compiled by Dr.

Bruce Fife in his books and other researchers in the field, including this author.

- They support healthy cholesterol formation in the liver. This high-density lipoprotein (HDL) is the kind of cholesterol we want and that is essential to healthy hormone production. HDL cholesterol is not implicated in calcification diseases like coronary heart disease. Coconut products have never been implicated in any coronary diseases. The saturated fat that comes from cooked animal products (cooked meat and pasteurized dairy milk and cheese) can actually be dangerous because they are so sticky that they become a growth medium for calcium-forming organisms that hook onto them like barnacles and then plug up the capillaries and eventually the entire cardiovascular system. In addition, factory-farmed animal products (meat, chicken, cheese, milk, etc.) are themselves already contaminated with calcium-forming organisms, thus their consumption increases calcification rates in our bodies. Calcification inevitably becomes the main contributing factor in nearly every chronic disease condition.

The following benefits may be derived from consuming fresh, young, wild coconut water:

- An excellent nutrition source for infants.
- Great for rehydration.
- Contains organic compounds possessing growth-promoting properties—coconut is excellent for improving muscle size and general physical growth in children.
- Cooling effects on the body (reverses pitta aggravation in the Ayurvedic system of medicine).
- Topical application on the body helps soothe and even prevent skin eruptions and rashes.

- The presence of organic sodium and albumin in coconut water makes it a good drink for cholera cases.
- Helps to calm urinary tract infections (applying my Ormus Gold product topically is recommended for urinary tract infections).
- An excellent tonic for all ages.
- Effective in helping to alleviate the pain of kidney and urethral stones. Coconut water helps to fight nanobacteria and the production of bad calcium in the kidneys.
- Used as blood plasma substitute because it is sterile, does not produce heat, does not destroy red blood cells, and is readily accepted by the body.

Medium-Chain Fatty Acids (MCFAs)

Fats are chains of carbon atoms of varying lengths surrounded by hydrogen. The arrangement of hydrogen around a carbon chain determines its saturation. The more hydrogen, the more saturation and the more stable the molecule.

The length of the carbon chain in fat determines many of its properties. Coconut oil is a saturated fat, but it consists primarily of medium chain fatty acids (MCFAs, sometimes called medium-chain triglycerides, or MCTs) of eight to twelve carbon atoms in length. Some saturated fatty acids in meats, for example, range in length from fourteen to twenty-four carbon atoms while some of those in butter and vinegar range in length from two to six carbon atoms in length.

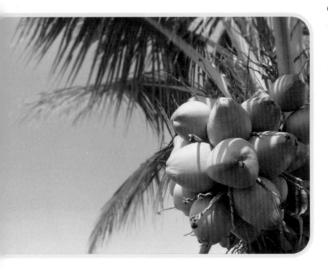

The shorter MCFA chains require less energy and fewer enzymes to digest. In most people, coconut cream and oil can be emulsified during digestion without excessively burdening the liver or gall bladder. Thus, coconut cream and oil provide more energy, more quickly, than other fat sources. Many individuals who suffer from poor digestion—and especially liver or gall bladder trouble—can benefit from consuming coconut oil in place of other oils.

MCFA Immune System-Enhancing Properties

I use medium chain triglycerides or organic coconut oil as sources of antimicrobial fatty acids.

—Udo Erasmus, author of *Fats That Heal, Fats That Kill*

The MCFAs in coconut cream and coconut oil possess incredible health-giving properties. Coconut cream and coconut oil contain the following MCFAs:

Caprylic acid (C-8)
Capric acid (C-10)
Lauric acid (C-12)
Myristic acid (C-14)

All these demonstrate antiviral, antimicrobial, and antifungal properties. Lauric acid has the greatest antiviral activity. Caprylic acid is the most potent yeast-fighting substance.

MCFAs disrupt the lipid membranes of viruses, bacteria, yeast, and fungi. Lipid-coated viruses and bacteria contain lipids in their membranes that are similar to those in MCFAs. MCFAs confuse microbes and viruses because they can no longer calibrate the location of their membranes in the presence of coconut oil. This causes them to spill their genetic contents and become easy prey for white blood cells to consume.

Those who suffer from candida or other fungal conditions can benefit from coconut oil. Some forms of psoriasis are actually skin infections caused by fungi in combination with calcium-forming organisms (micro-shell-forming nanobacteria). These infections can be helped by using coconut oil topically.

Cholesterol

Most information circulating in the mass media about saturated fat and cholesterol is inaccurate. Saturated fats have been the target of a host of hostile propaganda. This propaganda claims that saturated fats lead to clogging of the arteries, when, in reality, arterial plaque is directly related to the consumption of rancid unsaturated fat (vegetable oil such as corn oil and partially hydrogenated soybean oil)—as well as foreign LDL cholesterol (derived from eating animal products) and bad calcium formed by infectious micro-shell-forming nanobacteria.

Blackburn et al. (1988) reviewed the published literature of "coconut oil's effect on serum cholesterol and atherogenesis" and concluded that when "fed physiologically with other fats or adequately supplemented with linoleic acid, coconut oil is a neutral fat in terms of atherogenicity."

Coconut oil contains virtually no cholesterol and actually helps normalize cholesterol levels. It outperforms cold-pressed olive oil in this regard. Coconut-eating cultures in the tropics have consistently lower cholesterol levels than people in the U.S.

The cholesterol-normalizing properties of coconut oil are a direct result of its ability to stimulate thyroid function. In the presence of adequate thyroid hormone, cholesterol (specifically LDL cholesterol) is converted by enzymatic processes to necessary anti-aging steroids, progesterone, DHEA, and pregnenolone. These substances are required to help prevent heart disease, senility, obesity, cancer, and other diseases associated with aging and degeneration.

In his books, Dr. Raymond Peat (a leading researcher in the field of hormones) details that coconut products, when regularly added to a balanced diet, lower cholesterol to normal by promoting their conversion into pregnenolone. Pregnenolone is also the precursor to many hormones including progesterone. Dr. Peat recommends that women with hormone imbalances increase their pregnenolone levels.

Pregnenolone is a major factor that gives coconut products their beautifying qualities. Pregnenolone improves circulation in the skin, gives the face a lift, restores sagging skin, and reduces bags under the eyes by promoting the contractions of musclelike cells. Pregnenolone counters fatigue, enhances the memory, protects the nerves from stress, and has anti-anxiety properties.

Antioxidants

As a derivative of the coconut, pregnenolone is an antioxidant. Coconut oil itself appears to have strong antioxidant properties since the oil is highly stable and reduces our need for vitamin E, whereas unsaturated vegetable oils such as cottonseed, soybean, and corn oil deplete vitamin E.

Research findings indicate that coconut oil appears to double the body's ability to use antioxidant, omega-3 fatty acids. Because of this, I recommend that individuals take omega-3 containing oils (flaxseed oil, hempseed oil, krill oil, algae oil, etc.) with coconut oil.

Blood Sugar

For those of us who use coconut cream or oil consistently, one of the most noticeable changes is the ability to go for several hours without eating, and to feel hungry without having symptoms of hypoglycemia and erratic blood-sugar levels. Erratic blood sugar swings stress the system, thus activating the adrenal glands (low blood sugar is a signal for the release of adrenal hormones).

Shifting to coconut cream or oil as a fat source normalizes blood-sugar levels, increases energy, decreases the stress on our system, and thus reduces our need for the adrenal hormones. Removing the effects of adrenal stress alleviates dark circles from around the eyes.

The Thyroid Gland and Weight Loss

Dr. Peat describes that in the 1940s, farmers attempted to use coconut fat to fatten their animals, yet they found it made the animals lean and active—not the effect they were looking for. The farmers wanted to fatten their animals for slaughter and thus, within ten years, chose to give their animals soy and corn feed. Soy and corn feed slow the thyroid, causing animals to get fat without eating much food.

Cooked, unsaturated oils (corn oil, safflower oil, canola oil, soy margarine, etc.) suppress the metabolism, contributing to hypothyroidism (and weight gain). This occurs because cooked, unsaturated oils not only suppress our tissue's response to the thyroid hormone, but also suppress the transport of the hormone on the thyroid-transport protein.

Consuming coconut products regularly helps restore thyroid function and actually increases the metabolic rate leading to weight loss. Those who are taking artificial thyroid medication must be cautious in coming off that drug. Thyroid medication strongly influences metabolism. Please consult with your holistic physician if you undergo a program to wean yourself from thyroid medication.

The Skin and Nervous System

Coconut oil is generally antiviral. Coconut cream may be antiviral (with the exception of herpes viruses) due to its MCFA content. The pulverizing of coconut cream in a conch or stone-grinder makes the arginine amino acid, and probably several other elements, more bioavailable. When coconut is used as a cream rather than an oil, the herpes family of viruses (when an infection is deep enough in the nervous system) can derive enough food out of the coconut cream to multiply—especially during a stressful time. This is actually true of every nut butter that we know of (almond butter, cashew butter, etc.) and is also true of chocolate—especially when it is cooked and conched (liquefied and stirred). Skin eruptions and breakouts may not occur every time, but there is a distinctive link between outbreaks and this class of foods. Therefore, coconut cream along with all nut butters are not recommended if one is suffering from herpes. If herpes is a problem for you, please obtain, study, and immediately act on my *LongevityNOW Program* (see www.thebestdayever.com) where a system is detailed on how to eliminate herpes from being a problem in your life. The *LongevityNOW Program* also provides tools to lower dangerous calcification levels in the body and restore elastic, healthy joints, organs, skin, and connective tissue.

After a bottle of unsaturated oil (corn oil, safflower oil, canola oil, soy margarine, etc.) has been opened several times, a few drops typically dribble onto the outside of the bottle. These drops become very sticky and difficult to wash off. Once inside the body, this characteristic of rancid oil leads to wrinkles, "liver spots" on the skin, and lesions in the brain, heart, blood vessels, and eyes. As cooked, unsaturated (vegetable) oil increases in the diet, the rate of oxidative damage increases, leading to aged, damaged organs such as the liver, heart, and skin.

Rancid fats and oils found in everyday commercial lotions and creams are absorbed through the skin and negatively affect the connective tissues. They provide temporary relief from dry skin, but eventually weaken the skin over time. Generally, the more standard commercial lotions and creams that one uses, the worse the skin becomes. In his book *The Coconut Oil Miracle*, Bruce Fife, ND, writes, "Studies show that dry skin contains a higher content of unsaturated fatty acids (60 percent) compared to normal skin (49 percent). The best oil to use is one that doesn't create free radicals. Saturated fats fit that requirement."

In my opinion, coconut oil is an essential lotion. I use this coconut oil as a lotion after sunbathing to help create and hold onto a beautiful tan. Even when not sunbathing, you can rub it into your hands, shoulders, and neck, and even into your gums. Coconut oil has a pleasant odor and provides a radiance to the skin.

What about coconut meat and the coconut oil in coconut? The young, wild flesh of the coconut (spoon-meat) is the best builder of male sexual fluids of any food. In the Ayurvedic understanding, it takes thirty-five days to refine food all the way from its basic state when you first chew it up, all the way into your blood, your bones, the lymphatic fluid, essentially through all the seven different levels of transformations, until it reaches the final stage, which is your reproductive fluid. Coconut spoon-meat can get there in one day. It is already in that state.

In women, the young spoon-meat can be instantly developed into breast milk. Coconut and coconut products in general are valuable foods for pregnancy, post-pregnancy recovery, and breast-feeding.

What to Look For . . .

Coconut Product Types

Wild coconuts: Available in most tropical locations worldwide.

Thai hybrid coconuts

Brown coconuts: Select brown, hairy coconuts by looking at the three holes on one side of the coconut. If there is mold on any of the three holes, select a different coconut. Always purchase coconuts free of mold.

Coconut water: Use the cardboard container products rather than aluminum container products. Aluminum is toxic and has been implicated in causing Alzheimer's disease.

Coconut oil: Preferably select coconut oil in amber glass. Avoid plastic containers if possible. Plastics may leach into coconut oil due to the oil's solvent properties.

Coconut cream (sometimes called coconut butter): Made from stone-ground or conched copra or coconut flakes, this product still contains the coconut fiber. Coconut cream is thick and has a cream cheese type of taste. It packs a lot of nutrition and fewer calories than other nut butters.

Coconut flakes (shredded copra)

Coconut powder

Coconut Oil in Dark Glass

As with any oil, all coconut butter/oil that you use should be cold-pressed and packaged in dark glass bottles. All butters and oils are light sensitive. Dark, amber glass containers keep damaging spectrums of light from reaching the oil.

Coconut oil in dark glass is very stable and can be kept in a cupboard at room temperature. It can be refrigerated after opening, but this is not required to ensure freshness. It can remain stable for over two years (some people suggest up to five years) with proper storage—no light, heat, or oxygen. In *The Coconut Oil Miracle,* Fife also tells us:

> According to Leigh Broadhurst, PhD, a scientist at the USDA Human Nutrition Research Center in Beltville, Maryland, saturated fatty acids are 300 or more times more resistant to oxidation than alpha-linolenic acid (flaxseed oil). In other words, coconut oil will remain fresh 300 times longer than flaxseed oil. For instance, to equal the amount of oxidative damage that occurs in flaxseed oil in just 30 minutes of processing, coconut oil would have to be subjected to the same conditions for 150 continuous hours—that's over six days.

Repairing and nourishing the skin and our other organs with coconut oil should be done by both eating coconut oil and massaging it into the skin.

Coconut oil reverses the tissue-damaging process by displacing sticky, cooked oil from tissues and providing fat-soluble vitamins, minerals, and super-nutrition factors (especially pregnenolone) directly to the damaged tissue.

Coconut oil has been used as a skin moisturizer for thousands of years. It is ideal for dry, rough, and wrinkled skin. Because it consists mostly of MCFAs, it is easily absorbed by the skin. It prevents stretch marks and lightens existing ones. It is an excellent lip balm. Its antiseptic elements keep the skin young, healthy, and relatively free from infections. All these factors make coconut oil ideal for massage and massage therapists.

How to Use Coconut Products

Any young coconut can be chopped open with a machete or butcher knife. Be sure to keep all your fingers well clear of the chopping blade. You can drink the water with a straw (glass straws are wonderful) and then the young white flesh on the inside of the coconut is ready for consumption. To get the white flesh, cut the nut in half and spoon out the fresh, young spoon-meat. Quarter the remaining coconut husk (split each side of the inner coconut bowl) in order to avoid creating small bowls that can pool water where mosquitoes can proliferate (this is important if you live in the tropics). Coconut husks are excellent for compost and for campfire burning.

Coconut flesh can be added to coconut water and blended. This blend is called coconut milk, as it has a solid white appearance.

Coconut flesh can also be dried and/or dehydrated with herbs and spices and prepared like a "jerky."

Coconut cream is a thick, rich, nutritious snack for children and adults. Adults can consume 2–4 tablespoons of coconut cream daily, either straight or blended into a favorite beverage (tea, smoothie, elixir) or mixed as a snack with other superfoods (goji berries, marine phytoplankton, spirulina, bee pollen, etc.). Coconut cream can be used to create delicious chocolates, elixirs, and desserts.

Coconut oil can be eaten straight, blended into a salad dressing, or added into any kind of smoothie (superfood, chocolate, fruit) you wish. The recommended daily intake is one to four tablespoons (a therapeutic dose consists of at least three tablespoons daily).

Try drinking coconut water with a superfood protein (spirulina, blue-green algae, chlorella, hempseed protein, etc.), which you may find gives you the long-lasting, stable energy you are looking for. Coconut water is a flavorful, excellent delivery system for powdered superfood protein sources and is the ideal base liquid for nearly any smoothie or shake you could make.

Coconut Fat

Coconut fat is made by heating mature, dried coconut flakes in hot water, which extracts the coconut oil and aromatic elements. When refrigerated, the coconut fat will rise to the top and separate out of the water. This is another way, other than pressing the copra, to remove the oil from the coconut. This type of coconut oil is generally considered superior to the common coconut oil used for cosmetic uses.

Cooking

One of the greatest pieces of information one could derive from this book is to only and exclusively use coconut oil for all cooking needs. Coconut oil is the most stable (of any known butter/oil) at high temperatures (up to 170 degrees Fahrenheit). Therefore, if one is going to heat or cook any food, coconut oil should be the only butter/oil used. This means using coconut oil for cooking in place of butter, margarine, canola oil, corn oil, or safflower oil. Unlike all of these fats/oils, coconut oil does not form polymerized oils or dangerous trans-fatty acids because it is a completely saturated fat. Due to its complete saturation, coconut is superior to even olive oil as a cooking oil.

Coconut Oil as Topical and Erotic Oil

Coconut oil is a great topical oil. Coconut oil and its MCFAs naturally help eliminate unhealthy, toxic bacteria from the skin and simultaneously foster a skin environment where friendly organisms can live happily. This results in beautiful, healthy, soft, youthful skin. Coconut oil can be applied to most areas of the body, with the exception of the fine pores on the face and scalp.

Coconut oil, like cacao butter, is also a fantastic erotic oil. The smell and taste of this oil enhance sexual intercourse. Its antiviral, antimicrobial properties are generally not strong enough to protect from sexually transmitted diseases (STDs) so for new relationships, condoms and other appropriate protection from STDs should be used, but for long-term monogamous relationships, coconut oil is a great choice. Coconut oil should be used with polyurethane condoms or a natural skin condom. Latex condoms should not be used, because coconut oil can dissolve latex.

You can make a homemade oil by mixing cacao butter and coconut oil 50-50, using a slight amount of heat to liquefy them both. Try this on your skin for magical skin nutrition.

Teeth

Take a teaspoon of coconut oil and apply it to your (or your child's) gums and teeth to kill germs in the mouth and help normalize oral pH. Coconut oil can help protect your teeth. Coconut oil contributes to healthy biofilms in the mouth.

Storing Coconut Oil and Coconut Cream

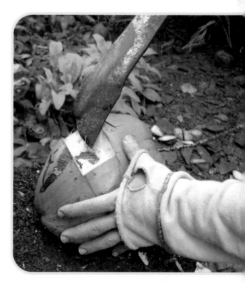

High-quality coconut oil is very stable and requires no refrigeration. Coconut cream is slightly less antimicrobial and therefore should be refrigerated for added freshness.

A Note of Caution about Coconut Water

Fresh coconut water is not a replacement for drinking water. Although coconut water can diminish excessive water needs, regular drinking water should still be consumed. In addition, coconut water is best avoided in individuals with hyperkalaemia (excessive potassium) conditions such as renal failure, acute adrenal insufficiency, low urine output due to haemolysis following blood transfusions, or in those individuals who have just been treated with a snakebite serum, in which potassium may be unusually high.

Coconut Recipes

Goji Coconut Balls

by Sandy B. "Chocolate Face"

    1 cup shredded coconut flakes
    1/2 cup coconut oil
    11/2 cup raw cashews
    11/4 cup hempseed
    1/2 cup goji berry extract powder
    11/2 cup goji berries
    1 cup tocotrienols
    21/2 tbsps. raw honey
    1 pinch or two of Celtic sea salt

Grind seeds and nuts separately in a coffee grinder, then add the remaining ingredients to a high-speed blender or food processor and blend until turned into a mush. Roll this mush into balls and refrigerate.

Coconut Cream Dream

Combine the following in a blender—and fly!

    inner flesh from 2–3 whole, young Thai coconuts
    water from 1 young Thai coconut

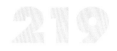

2 handfuls raw cashews (unsoaked)

2 vanilla beans (scrape out inner powder, do not use the outer skin)

3 tbsp. tocotrienols

2 tbsp. raw Manuka honey (or your other favorite raw honey)

1/2 cup shredded, dried coconut flakes, blended into a powder

1/3–1/2 cup coconut oil

cut pieces of one Sacred Chocolate™ bar

Pour the blended thick cream into a bowl, add Sacred Chocolate™ pieces, and enjoy to your heart's delight!

Parfait variation: Pour an abundance of cream over a bowl of your favorite fresh, seasonal, chopped fruit. I especially enjoy the following (combine according to the artistic genius of your taste buds): strawberries, blueberries, blackberries, raspberries, mangoes, apricots, peaches, persimmons, and pineapple.

Durian de la Creme

2 whole young Thai coconuts (use both the inner flesh and water)

2 "pods" (about 2 big handfuls) of durian (fresh or frozen)

2–3 tsp. mesquite powder

1–2 vanilla beans (scrape out inner powder, do not use the outer skin)

2–3 tbsp. tocotrienols

1 tbsp. raw NoniLand™ honey or Manuka honey

1/4–1/2 tsp. cinnamon

1/4 tsp. fresh ground nutmeg (optional)

Combine these ingredients in a blender, pour into glasses, and experience the true bliss of raw living!

For a frosty, ice-creamy treat, stick the glasses in the freezer for as long as you can possibly hold out (maximum 4 hours), and enjoy!

Coconut Jerkylicious

Mix the following ingredients in a large bowl (feel free to adjust proportions to taste):

  1/4 cup curry powder (or you can try your favorite Italian herb
    seasoning blend)

  2 tbsp. raw honey (or yacon syrup)

  1 tsp. Celtic sea salt

  1/3–1/2 cup coconut oil, melted

  Optional: 1–2 tsp. cayenne powder (if you like it spicy!)

Pour out the water into a separate container and scoop out the inner flesh from 4 young Thai coconuts. Mix the flesh into the bowl with the combined ingredients and let marinate for at least 2 hours (overnight is best) in the refrigerator.

Once it has marinated, remove the soaked coconut flesh from the bowl and place on a dehydrator tray or a stove sheet. Dehydrate the treated coconut flesh in a dehydrator or stove. Dry at no hotter than 120 degrees F until the coconut has achieved a chewy, jerky-like consistency.

This treat is great alone as a snack or served atop salad.

One Minute Superfood Blood Plasma Transfusion

  water from 2 young Thai coconuts

  2 tsp. powdered marine phytoplankton

  2 tsp. blue-green algae (Crystal Manna, E3Live™ Flakes, etc.)

  1 squirt Dr. Patrick Flanagan's Crystal Energy

Pour coconut water into a glass, add superfoods, and stir your way to super rejuvenation and full-body hydration.

Heavenly Coconut Milk

Blend the following, and then strain through a nut-milk bag or cheesecloth:

> water from 2–3 young Thai coconuts
>
> 1/2 cup hempseed

Pour strained liquid back into the blender and add:

> insides of 1–2 raw vanilla beans (not the outside skin)
>
> 1 tbsp. mesquite powder
>
> 1 small pinch Celtic sea salt
>
> 1–2 tsp. coconut oil
>
> 1 tbsp. (or less) raw NoniLand™ honey (or other favorite raw honey) or yacon syrup
>
> 1 tbsp. tocotrienols
>
> 1 squirt Dr. Patrick Flanagan's Crystal Energy

Pour and enjoy pure decadence in a cup!

Coconut Spice Medley

> 2 cups shredded, dried coconut flakes
>
> 1 thumb-sized piece of fresh ginger
>
> 1 thumb-sized piece of fresh turmeric
>
> 1 tsp. crushed chili powder
>
> 1/4 cup lime juice
>
> 2 tbsp. raw NoniLand™ honey (or other favorite raw honey) or yacon syrup

Grate the hard coconut, turmeric, and ginger into a bowl. Add lime juice, chili, and honey.

Enjoy as a salad topping, a spread on your favorite raw flax crackers or bread, inside a raw veggie wrap, served atop fresh vegetables, or as a dip.

Bavarian Custard

Recipe by Elaina Love

> 2 cups young coconut milk
>
> 1/2 cup coconut water
>
> 2 tbsp. orange juice (1/2 orange)
>
> 1/8 tsp. Himalayan crystal salt
>
> 1 pinch (~1/8 tsp.) powdered turmeric for color
>
> 1 vanilla bean (scraped)
>
> 1 tsp. vanilla extract
>
> 1/4 tsp. almond extract
>
> 1/4 cup agave nectar or more to taste (raw honey or yacon syrup can also be substituted if desired)
>
> 1 tbsp. non-GMO soy lecithin
>
> 1 tbsp. coconut oil or coconut butter

Blend on high until the mixture is creamy. Refrigerate until cool and serve. Serves 4.

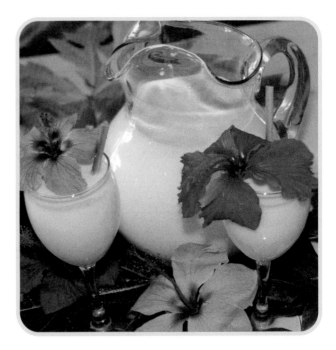

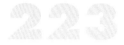
Vanilla Coconut Ice Cream

Recipe by Elaina Love

  2 cups raw almonds

  3 cups spring water

  1/2 cup coconut oil

  1/4 cup packed Irish moss, after soaking 3–8 hours and rinsing well

  1 cup agave nectar (or your favorite raw honey)

  1/4 tsp. vanilla powder

  2 tsp. vanilla extract

  1/4 tsp. Himalayan salt crystals

Blend the almonds with water to make a thick almond cream. Strain the mixture through a nut-milk bag and store the pulp for another recipe. Blend 1 cup of the almond milk with the Irish moss until very smooth. Add the remainder of ingredients and blend until smooth. Pour into a freezable container and let freeze overnight. Let thaw about 5 minutes before serving.

Variations: Replace water with nut milk or with any flavored teas such as peppermint, orange, or berry. You can also blend in 1/4 cup raw cacao powder or 1/2 cup of fruit such as berries.

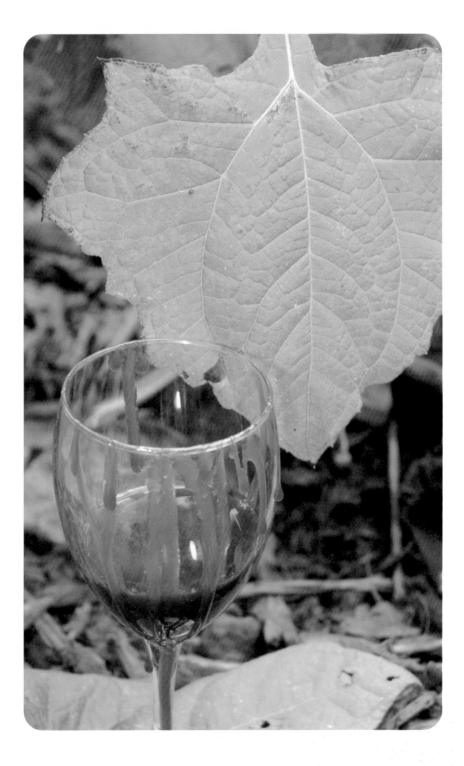

Honorable Mentions

In alphabetical order:

Açai
Camu Camu Berry
Chlorella
Incan Berries
Kelp
Noni
Yacon

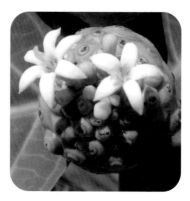

These "honorable mentions" are each superfoods in their own right that for reasons (strictly my own) did not make my top ten list. They might make yours. Read about them. Eat them. Explore these and other superfoods and have The Best Day Ever!

Açai: Ancient Amazonian Antioxidant

(Pronounced ah-SAH'-ee)

Açai is a little blue (sometimes purple) berry that originated in the Amazon rainforest of Brazil. Considered to be one of the most powerful and nutritious superfoods on the planet, açai has been used for centuries by the natives of Brazil for its legendary health properties.

Açai palm trees (*Euterpe badiocarpa* and *Euterpe oleracea*) can grow to heights of fifty to eighty feet tall. Four to eight individual trees often grow from one seed.

The açai palm tree can be found in the tropical flood plains and river-bank regions of the Amazon basin in Brazil, South America. A very climate-specific plant, açai is only found growing in tropical regions near the equator. Because the equatorial tropics are one of the harshest and most UV ray–intense zones of our planet, in order to protect itself from the sun, the açai berry must produce high amounts of its own UV protective "sunscreen"—the substances we know as "antioxidants."

The açai palm tree has small, brownish-purple flowers and produces large bunches of edible berries. When ripe, the berries are dark blue-purple and about the size of a large blueberry. They contain a thin layer of delicious, edible pulp surrounding a large seed. Once the açai fruits become ripe and are harvested, the thin fruit pulp is processed into more concentrated forms (such as powder) by a variety of methods, depending on the supplier.

This antioxidant-rich Amazonian berry has recently gotten a lot of mainstream attention (it made Oprah Winfrey's Top 10 Superfoods List) due to its astounding health benefits as a potent, longevity-promoting superfood.

Benefits and Key Discoveries about Açai

- Contains high levels of essential fatty acids (omega-3, omega-6) as well as omega-9 and monounsaturated oleic acid. Oleic acid is a beautifying oil.
- Super rich in blue-pigmented antioxidants. The antioxidant content of açai berries is truly remarkable. Açai has one of the highest known ORAC (Oxygen Radical Absorption Capacity) values in the world, earning it the well-deserved "superfruit" title. (The ORAC assay is a standard measure of antioxidant concentration.) Phenols and anthocyanins (an extraordinary 320 mg per 100 grams), the potent antioxidants responsible for the berry's appealing dark blue to purple color, play a critical role in neutralizing free radicals (aggressive oxygen) within the body, thus promoting longevity. In recent tests, açai scored an ORAC value of 185. In comparison, red grapes came in at 11, blueberries at 32, and pomegranate at 105.

- According to recent research, açai appears to help regenerate and produce stem cells. Stem cells are the embryos of all cells. They help us rejuvenate and heal faster by becoming any cell that is needed within our bodies. For example, a stem cell can become a connective tissue cell, a white blood cell, a muscle cell, or a nerve cell—anything we need. The more we produce stem cells, the more we regenerate, and the longer we can live.
- Contains large amounts of plant sterols, especially beta sitosterol. Plant sterols are naturally occurring compounds within certain plants that have been found to inhibit the absorption of excessive animal-food-based cholesterol within the GI tract.
- Contains nineteen different amino acids necessary for building healthy proteins throughout the body.
- Excellent source of dietary fiber (aids in digestion).
- Low-glycemic level. Açai is low in sugar.
- Rich in minerals and vitamins, especially calcium, phosphorus, beta-carotene, and vitamin E.
- Fights cancer: A recent University of Florida (UF) Study, published in the *Journal of Agricultural and Food Chemistry*, showed extracts from açai berries triggered a self-destruct response in up to 86 percent of leukemia cells tested, said Stephen Talcott, an assistant professor with UF's Institute of Food and Agricultural Sciences. "Açai berries are already considered one of the richest fruit sources of antioxidants," Talcott said. "This study was an important step toward learning what people may gain from using beverages, dietary supplements, or other products made with the berries."

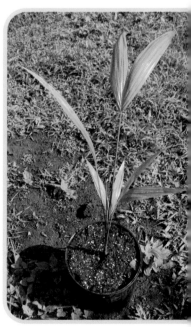

All of these benefits add up to a superfood that is a great natural energy booster, helps enhance nerve and brain function, promotes a healthy cardiovascular system, supports the creation of healthy, smooth skin, improves endurance and muscular development, assists with digestive health, increases the power of our immune system, and allows our body to more swiftly rejuvenate.

What to Look for in Açai

- Organic: Always select organic superfoods whenever possible. Organic foods are grown without chemical pesticides and artificial fertilizers.
- Fair Trade: Fair trade guarantees fair wages for workers, improving their opportunities for better health-care, housing, and education. By choosing fair-trade açai, you are directly contributing to the livelihood of rainforest communities.
- The highest nutrition content is in the açai fruit skin, so if you are considering any açai product you would want as much of the skin as possible in the product.
- Proper freeze drying (if you cannot obtain açai fresh): If you can confirm that the açai powder is made from açai berries that were freeze-dried within hours of being picked, you can expect antioxidant levels ranging from 30 to 50 percent of levels found in the pulp of fresh açai berries.

Two of my favorite açai brands are *Sambazon* and *Amazon Thunder.*

Camu Camu Berry: Vitamin C Sun King

There is no doubt that ascorbic acid [Vitamin C] is required for the synthesis of collagen in the bodies of human beings and other animals. One of the important functions of collagen is its service in strengthening the intercellular cement that holds the cells of the body together in various tissues. It is not unlikely that part of the effectiveness of vitamin C against the common cold, influenza, and other viral diseases can be attributed to this strengthening effect, and in this way preventing or hindering the motion of the virus particles through the tissues and into the cells.

    —Linus Pauling, *Vitamin C, the Common Cold, and the Flu*

Camu camu (*Myrciaria dubia*) is a bush native to South American tropical rainforests that produces a fruit containing more vitamin C than any other known botanical source (for comparison: a fresh camu camu berry may contain up to 4 percent vitamin C, whereas a lemon may contain up to 0.5 percent vitamin C). Some estimate that camu camu berries have thirty times as much vitamin C as oranges.

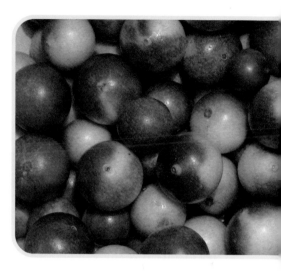

Consider the words of Dr. James Duke, USDA scientist and author of *The Green Pharmacy:* "I take vitamin C for colds ... I prefer to get mine from camu camu, the amazing Amazonian fruit that has the world's highest vitamin C content."

Indigenous Amazonian peoples traditionally pick the camu camu berries in season, dry them, and use them medicinally for the rest of the year. This purplish-red berry becomes light beige in color when dried and powdered.

The camu camu berry is an excellent source of calcium, phosphorus, potassium, iron, the amino acids serine, valine, and leucine, as well as small amounts of the vitamins thiamine, riboflavin, and niacin. Camu camu berry is usually available in a dried, powdered form. The powder tastes delicious and tangy. Traditionally, camu camu has been used to:

- support the immune system,
- maintain excellent eyesight,
- create beautiful skin,
- ward off viral infections,
- support strong collagen, tendons, and ligaments,
- decrease inflammation,
- improve respiratory (lung) health,
- help maintain optimal clarity of mind in times of stress and anxiety, and
- especially support the functions of the brain, eyes, heart, liver, and skin.

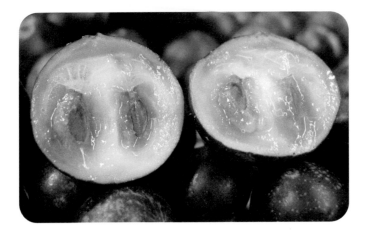

In a comparative study of hundreds of botanicals, ranked in order of effectiveness for various health conditions, camu camu was placed by Dr. Duke among hundreds of herbs as follows*:

Antimutagenic	#4
Antioxidant	#4
Antiviral	#6
Asthma	#1
Atherosclerosis	#1
Cataracts	#1
Colds	#1
Depression	#2
Edema	#1
Gingivitis/Periodontal disease	#1
Glaucoma	#1
Hepatitis	#1
Infertility	#1
Migraine headaches	#1
Osteoarthritis	#1
Painkiller	#1
Parkinson's disease	#1

*Note: This comparative study's results are not FDA approved. We make no specific claim as to the camu camu berry's medicinal properties.

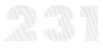
Recommended Dosage

1 level tbsp. (3 grams) of camu camu berry powder per person per day. One can increase dosage with time. Diarrhea symptoms indicate excessive intake.

How to Use Camu Camu Berry Powder

Add one level tbsp. (3 grams) or more to juices, smoothies, raw ice creams, raw desserts, or simply to your drinking water. As a natural vitamin C source, this product may be used in conjunction with MSM powder to rejuvenate collagen.

Chlorella: Green Pigment of Your Imagination

Chlorella is a single-celled, water-grown algae that consists primarily of a nucleus and a large amount of directly available chlorophyll, a nutrient vital to the health of our bodies. Chlorella is a whole food, as it is extremely rich in vitamins, minerals, amino acids, essential fatty acids, polysaccharides, and a host of other beneficial compounds. Chlorella supports the function of the brain and liver, improves digestion and elimination, helps regenerate the body (especially in cases of degeneration), detoxifies the body, protects against radiation, relieves inflammation, supports healthy weight loss, enhances the immune system, and, overall, accelerates the healing process.

Both scientific documentation and reliable anecdotal reports indicate that chlorella is effective in reducing the symptoms of numerous types of cancers, diabetes, low blood sugar, arthritis, AIDS, candida, pancreatitis, liver cirrhosis, hepatitis, peptic ulcers, viral and bacterial infections, anemia, and multiple sclerosis.

Highest Known Chlorophyll Content

Chlorella gets its name from the rich quantity of chlorophyll it possesses. Chlorella contains more chlorophyll per gram than any other plant. Chlorophyll is one of the greatest food substances for rejuvenating the blood and cleansing the bowels and other elimination systems such as the liver.

Green microalgae are the highest sources of chlorophyll in the plant world. And of all the green algae studied so far, chlorella has the highest, often ranging from 3 to 5 percent pure natural chlorophyll.

Detoxifies the Body and Supports Optimum Liver Function

Chlorella is considered to be a first-class detoxifying agent, capable of removing alcohol from the liver and/or clearing heavy metals, certain pesticides, herbicides, and polychlorbiphenyls (PCBs) from the body's tissues. In Japan, interest in chlorella has focused largely on this superfood's ability to remove or neutralize poisonous substances from the body that have accumulated due to environmental pollution and the ingestion of contaminated foods.

The Life Extension Foundation has cited many positive reports about chlorella from Japanese studies conducted after the nuclear catastrophes at Hiroshima and Nagasaki in 1945. In a report to the General Meeting of the Pharmaceutical Society of Japan on an early study in animals, Ichimura (1973) reported that chlorella (8 grams daily) increased the elimination of cadmium, threefold in feces and sevenfold in urine. Other researchers from Japan showed that chlorella helped detoxify uranium and lead.

Numerous research projects in the U.S. and Europe also indicate that chlorella can aid the body in breaking down persistent hydrocarbon and metallic toxins, specifically mercury (which is widely present in the bodies of many people in the form of toxic dental "amalgam" fillings), cadmium, arsenic, lead, DDT, and PCBs.

Chlorophyll also supports the optimum functioning and cleansing of the liver, which is the organ chiefly responsible for the general day-to-day detoxification of the body. A Japanese study showed that taking 4–6 grams of chlorella before consuming alcohol can prevent hangovers 96 percent of the time, even after a night of heavy drinking. Chlorella can also absorb toxins from the intestines, and, combined with its ability to favorably alter the bacterial flora content of the bowels, is able to help relieve chronic constipation and eliminate intestinal gas.

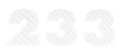
This detoxification of heavy metals and other chemical toxins in the blood will take three to six months, depending on how much chlorella a person is taking.

Immune Support for Whole-Body Rejuvenation

Chlorella extract is well known in the Japanese scientific community as a "biological response modifier." Studies have indicated that chlorella can provide critical benefits for the health of individuals with suppressed immune systems caused by chronic long-term illness or chemotherapy treatments. Research studies suggest that chlorella accelerates the recovery of developing immune system cells and restores the population of mature white blood cells. As best as we understand the process currently, white blood cells originate in the bone marrow as stem cells. From stem cells, white blood cells continue to multiply and grow as "colony-forming units." Cells increase in these colonies and mature into a variety of immune cells. In studies, chlorella accelerated the recovery of developing cells in colony-forming units and restored the population of mature white blood cells.

A newly available strain of chlorella contains a significant portion of the blue pigment phycocyanin that helps the body produce more stem cells. As we have seen with AFA blue-green algae and spirulina, when superfoods containing phycocyanin are consumed with superherbs such as reishi, maitake, or chaga mushroom the immune response is significantly improved.

Rats treated with the chemotherapy drug *cyclophosphamide* showed enhanced resistance against E. coli when given chlorella extract. Chlorella not only accelerated the recovery of white blood cell populations, but also enhanced their ability to respond and accumulate at the site of infection.

Supports the Immune System to Destroy Bacteria, Viruses, and Food-Borne Illnesses

Studies have shown that chlorella can increase the resistance to viral infections and enhance the ability to kill bacteria. For example, superoxide is a powerful weapon that white blood cells use to "blast away" bacteria. Given the same number of immune cells, the level of superoxide generated was one and a half times higher in mice receiving chlorella extract, thus enhancing the "killing ability" of those cells.

Another example: Cytomegalovirus is a herpes-type virus that can cause serious illness in patients treated with immune-suppressing drugs. Mice treated with chlorella extract prior to introduction of this virus survived lethal infection doses. Chlorella extract decreased virus replication in the organs by 58 to 65 percent. The extract increased the activity of gamma interferon, which stimulated natural killer cells to attack the virus.

Listeria monocytogene is a bacteria that has become a national concern due to increasing incidents of its presence in packaged foods. An infection can have lethal consequences for individuals with weakened immune systems. Chlorella extract significantly increased the resistance of mice infected with *Listeria monocytogenes,* producing a dose-dependent survival rate of 20 to 25 percent, while the control group not receiving chlorella extract had no survivors.

Chlorella Growth Factor

There is also another amazing property of chlorella called the "Chlorella Growth Factor" (CGF), which has baffled scientists throughout the world: chlorella quadruples itself every twenty hours, growing faster than any food crop known to man. When chlorella is ingested by the human body, it dramatically increases the rate of rebuilding and healing in tissues, multiplies the growth rate of the lactobacillus (beneficial bacteria) in the bowel, boosts the immune system, and fights free-radical damage. Chlorella also helps rebuild nerve tissue damage throughout the body and is excellent for treating degenerative brain and nerve disorders. This superfood is being used to help treat patients with Alzheimer's and Parkinson's disease.

> *Chlorella has been shown to improve immune function in people undergoing chemotherapy and/or radiation therapy. Chlorella increases macrophage activity, activates both T-cells and B-cells, and has shown antitumor effects. In addition, chlorellan, a substance found in chlorella, stimulates interferon production.*
>
> —Donald R. Yance, *Herbal Medicine, Healing & Cancer*

Highest Food Sources of RNA

It was previously believed that sardines were the highest food source of essential, longevity-enhancing RNA. This investigation was prompted when the oldest living American, age 135, was questioned about his diet, and replied that he ate canned sardines and crackers. Eating foods high in RNA/DNA provides material for the repair and production of human RNA/DNA. It is the breakdown of RNA and DNA in the cells that is believed to be a major factor in aging and degenerative diseases.

Research from Japan has shown *chlorella pyrenoidosa* is the highest-known food source of RNA. Chlorella has twenty times more RNA than sardines do (sardines contain 0.59 percent RNA, chlorella is 10 percent RNA). Bee pollen and royal jelly are also extraordinary sources of RNA and DNA.

Enzymes in Chlorella

Chlorella contains enzymes such as chlorophyllase and pepsin, which are two digestive enzymes. Enzymes perform a number of important functions in the body, especially relating to digestion. Chlorella that is freeze-dried or pasteurized may be lacking the benefit of chlorella's enzymes.

Causes Proliferation of "Good Bacteria"

Chlorella causes the lactobacilli bacteria in our stomachs to multiply at four times the normal rate. Taken with meals, chlorella helps provide very good digestion and more importantly, better assimilation of nutrients.

High Protein Content

Containing about 60 percent pure digestible protein, chlorella is one of the highest protein sources on the planet—far exceeding that of animal products like beef, chicken, and fish (18 to 30 percent protein).

Extremely Rich in Vitamins and Minerals

Chlorella is a whole food—it contains vitamins C and E, all of the B vitamins (including B12, which in chlorella may or may not be in a useable form for human metabolism), amino acids, folic acid, beta-carotene, lysine, and iodine. Chlorella is also extraordinarily rich in iron and calcium.

Naturally Rich in Essential Fatty Acids

Chlorella contains a greater quantity of fatty acids than either spirulina or wild blue-green. About 20 percent of these fatty acids are the artery-cleansing, omega-3, alpha-linolenic variety; perhaps this is one reason chlorella has been shown to be so effective in reducing cholesterol in the body and preventing atherosclerosis.

—Paul Pitchford, *Healing with Whole Foods*

One tablespoon of chlorella provides 320 percent of the RDA (Recommended Daily Allowance) of iron and 120 percent of the RDA of calcium.

How to Consume Chlorella

Chlorella greatly augments healthy digestion and overall digestive tract health. While it is almost impossible to take too much chlorella, it is best to introduce chlorella gradually into one's diet in order to allow the body to adapt to its deeply regenerative effects, especially on the digestive and intestinal systems.

Three grams per day is a good maintenance dosage of chlorella. With this amount, you will not notice significant changes but your body will get many of the nutrients it must have to function properly, such as amino acids (protein), vital minerals, vitamins, carbohydrates, and enzymes.

A person taking chlorella specifically for mercury detoxification would want to be taking around five to seven grams per day. This dosage is quite common, and at this level one will notice significant changes in digestion, energy, and overall health. One teaspoon of powder is equal to five grams (5,000 mg.)

Some people cannot tolerate chlorella, which might be due to a cellulase insufficiency. If you are unable to tolerate chlorella, it would be wise to consider using a different microalgae (spirulina, AFA blue-green, or marine phytoplankton) or adding a digestive enzyme supplement with cellulase in it to help digest the chlorella.

Incan Berries: Incan Trail Superfruit

Other Common Names for Incan Berries:

Aguaymanto berries
Golden berries
Peruvian gooseberries
Topotopo (Quechua)
Cuchuva (Aymara)
Motojobobo embolsado (Spanish)

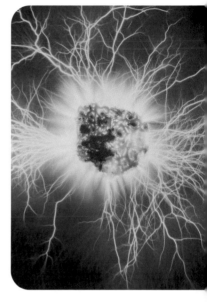

Andean crops have always been associated with improved health and longevity. Maca, yacon, and quinoa are some wonderful examples of food crops with high concentrations of phytonutrients that became staples for Andean cultures. Now the Incan berry *(Physalis peruviana)* emerges from its home in Peru as another example of an extraordinary food crop from the Andes.

Incan berries are generally considered among health enthusiasts to be the goji berry of South America, but Incan berries actually exceed goji berries in one area of nutrition: on average they contain 16 percent protein, compared to goji berries' 13 to 14 percent. This is an extraordinary level of protein for a fruit.

Incan berries grow wild in mineral-rich soils all over the Peruvian Andes. They are an ancient food, one of the "lost crops of the Incas," and highly prized in Peru. Incan berry bushes are one of the first plants to pioneer disturbed areas (the outskirts of towns, the fringes of housing developments, roads, etc.). Their robustness and adaptability confer adaptogenic qualities to the fruit. This means that when we eat Incan berries they help us adapt to different forms of physical, mental, and emotional stress.

Fresh Incan berries are protected by papery husks resembling Chinese lanterns. This thin, paperlike covering over the fruit—similar to that of a fresh tomatillo—has to be peeled away by hand before consuming the fruit or drying it.

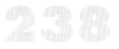

Harvest time of the Incan berry is concentrated from April to August. Most Incan berries in Peru are wild-grown native plants. However, some local farmers have developed orchards from the wild seeds.

With a pleasing, sweet flavor and a provocative tart tang, Incan berries add a delicious new dimension to our diet while working as an adaptogen to improve every aspect of our physical health. The flavor of Incan berries is midway between raw goji berries and wild-crafted barberries in sweetness, and their flavor has even been compared to dense, concentrated raspberries with a very distant hint of the Amazonian jungle peanut (probably due to their content of niacin). Incan berries may range in color from dark scarlet to sun-fire orange to yellow.

Typically, fresh berries from wild and cultivated berry farms are collected by hand and taken to a centralized processing farm cooperative. Here they are classified, cleaned, and prepared for later sun drying. Picking and drying these precious little berries is an intensely time-consuming job. In fact, one person takes a whole day to clean only about twenty-two pounds of fresh fruit! This is part of the reason why they are priced higher than other types of berries.

Once the fresh berries are ripe and cleaned, they are typically placed in sun dryers, and removed when the perfect level of moisture remains and there's still some delicious juiciness inside the berry. It takes approximately six pounds of fresh fruits to make one pound of dry berries. These dried, soft "giant raisins" are usually irregular in size 0.6–0.8 inches (1.6–2.0 cm). Once dried and packaged, Incan berries typically have a shelf life of one year.

Unique Benefits of the Incan Berry

- Incan berries can be used as ingredients in smoothies, fruit snacks, fruit bars, power bars, trail mixes, and much more. They add a delicious tangy flavor and chewy texture to all recipes.
- Incan berries are an excellent source of beta-carotene, vitamin C, thiamine, niacin, phosphorous, and protein. Remember, they exceed goji berries as one of the most protein-rich fruits at nearly 16 percent by dry weight.

- The small, chewable seeds inside the Incan berry have a mild laxative effect, making them an excellent food for intestinal health and regularity.
- Incan berries are also considered to be a good source of Secretory IgA, a plant antibody that helps support the immune system.
- Incan berries offer high levels of bioflavonoids, also known as vitamin P. Hundreds of studies on bioflavonoids have demonstrated they possess antisclerotic, antiviral, anticarcinogenic, anti-inflammatory, antihistamine, and antioxidant properties. This class of nutrients has been studied for its abilities to improve capillary strength while simultaneously preventing the buildup of atherosclerotic plaque in the blood vessels. Consuming foods rich in bioflavonoids plays a crucial role in detoxification and nutrient absorption. Improving the health of our capillaries is essential for the cardiovascular system and for those organs that require relatively high levels of nutrients and oxygen: the eyes, brain, and reproductive organs.
- Bioflavonoids also help enhance the benefit of vitamin C by improving its bioavailability and protecting this fragile nutrient from oxidation. It is clear that Incan berries and other foods rich in bioflavonoids contribute to a cascade of health benefits throughout the body.
- Incan berries also contain high levels of pectin. Long known for its ability to regulate the flow of food through the digestive tract, pectin also works to lower excess cholesterol levels, especially LDL cholesterol, which along with bioflavonoids prevents the accumulation of oxidized cholesterol in the blood vessels. Pectin is safe for those challenged by diabetes as it works to prevent surges in levels of blood glucose.

Suggested Uses for Incan Berries

From a simple trail mix to more exotic raw-food desserts, the festive colors of Incan berries help wake up any dish. Their distinctive balance of sweet and tart flavors make nutrient-dense Incan berries a great snack by themselves and in all sorts of combinations. Relax and enjoy a handful of Incan berries on their own while watching a film, or add them to goji berries and cacao nibs with hempseed in a trail mix, or blend them directly into an elixir and

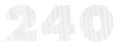

strain out the seeds, or sprinkle them on a salad. Incan berries are a low-glycemic, entirely guilt-free, wild superfood that are capable of working overtime to improve your health.

Incan berries love camu camu berries! Blend the two Peruvian berries, one from the Andes and one from the Amazon, together in any shake or sauce for a massive abundance of vitamin C. Blend up Incan berries, camu camu berry powder, water, lemons, Celtic sea salt, and NoniLand™ honey or yacon syrup for a fruity treat that will be sure to bring a smile to your face and a huge boost in immunity.

Improving the strength and flexibility of the capillaries with foods rich in bioflavonoids is vital for the health of the eyes, brain, and reproductive system. Hempseed, chia seeds, and powdered marine phytoplankton all offer concentrated sources of omega-3 fatty acids that work synergistically with bioflavonoids, allowing these organs to process information quickly and efficiently. Combine any of these foods with Incan berries for a tangy salad dressing with far-reaching health benefits.

Like most dried berries, Incan berries do not require refrigeration.

Kelp: Mineral Help-Gland of the Sea

Kelp is a sea vegetable (seaweed), which, like cacao, is extraordinarily rich in minerals, including alkaline minerals such as calcium and magnesium. Sufficient mineralization from proper nutrition has been known to normalize and calm behavior. A lack of proper mineral nutrition has been implicated in practically every symptom of poor health and emotionally extreme behavior.

Kelp is an especially rich source of potassium, iron, iodine, vitamin B6, riboflavin, and dietary fiber. It also contains glutamic acid, which enhances flavor and tenderizes fibrous foods. Phytochemicals in kelp have been shown to absorb and eliminate radioactive elements and heavy metal contaminants from our bodies.

Kelp is the most abundant, iodine-rich, sea vegetable. The iodine in kelp helps restore thyroid function, allowing one to improve metabolism and lose weight swiftly. The iodine and other minerals in kelp increase the mineral content of all the organs, allowing them to function more effectively. The better our organs function, the more readily they are able to throw off toxins and rejuvenate. Kelp also helps displace toxic minerals with healthy minerals (e.g., radioactive iodine with healthy iodine). Kelp is ideal as a seasoning substitute for salt.

The essential sugar (polysaccharide) known as xylose is also found in kelp. Xylose is antibacterial, antifungal, and helps prevent cancer of the digestive system.

Kelp contains another essential sugar known as fucose, which is antiviral, supports long-term memory, fights allergies, and guards against lung diseases. Fucose also helps alleviate cystic fibrosis, diabetes, cancer, and herpes.

Kelp is an excellent source of an additional essential sugar known as galactose, which improves memory, the absorption of good calcium, and the speedy healing of injuries.

The Role of Iodine in Health

Iodine itself is a poisonous gas, as are the related halogens chlorine, fluorine, and bromine. However, as with chlorine, the salts or negatively charged ions of iodine (iodides) are soluble in water, and in that form are essential in trace amounts to many life-forms. Most plants do not need iodine, but humans require it for the production of thyroid hormones that regulate the metabolic energy of the body and set the basal metabolic rate (BMR).

Iodine is well absorbed from the stomach into the blood. About 30 percent goes to the thyroid gland, depending on the need. Iodine is eliminated rapidly. Most of the remaining 70 percent is utilized by the immune system. What remains is filtered by the kidneys into the urine. Our bodies do not conserve iodine as they do iron, and we must obtain it regularly from the diet.

Iodine and Tin

Along with the element tin, iodine shares right- and left-sided cell receptors and is considered essential to human health. Tin is associated with iodine in the same way calcium is associated with magnesium, with tin supporting the adrenals, and iodine supporting the thyroid. The schizandra berry (a Chinese superherb) is the best-known source of the trace mineral tin.

Thyroid Gland Disorders

The thyroid is a small gland in the neck measuring about one inch across that lies just under the skin below the Adam's apple. The thyroid gland secretes thyroid hormones that control the speed of the body's metabolic rate.

To produce thyroid hormones, the thyroid gland needs iodine, an element contained in an ideal form in kelp. The thyroid gland traps iodine and processes it into thyroid hormones. As thyroid hormones are used up, some of the iodine contained in the hormones returns to the thyroid gland, where some is lost and the rest is recycled to produce more thyroid hormones.

As the thyroid stimulates energy production of the cellular mitochondria, it influences all body functions. Nerve health, bone formation, reproduction, the mineral condition of the skin, hair, nails, and teeth, as well as our speech and mental state are all influenced by thyroid. Thyroid and thus iodine also affect the conversion of carotene to vitamin A and of RNA to protein.

Iodine is a good example of a trace mineral whose deficiency creates an illness that is easily corrected by reintroducing it into the diet. Goiter, an enlargement of the thyroid gland, develops when the thyroid does not have enough iodine to manufacture hormones. As it increases its cell size to try to trap more iodine, the whole gland increases in size, creating a swelling in the neck. Even when a minor deficiency in the correct type of iodine occurs, a hypothyroid condition results, likely leading to fatigue and sluggishness, weight gain, and coldness of the body.

Noni: Polynesian Superfruit

Noni is the common name for *Morinda citrifolia,* a tropical tree native to Polynesia, especially to Tahiti and Hawaii. Polynesian *kahuna,* or traditional healers, have used noni fruits, leaves, stems, and roots in foods and beverages for the last two thousand years.

Noni fruit has a very distinctive odor and taste. Many people, especially when trying it fresh in the tropics, are repelled by the smell at first, but after eating the fruit over time come to love the taste. The health benefits definitely make this superfood well worth it!

The plant produces an irregular, lumpy, egg-shaped fruit reaching four or more inches in length. The ripe fruit has a strong, pungent odor. The seeds float due to inner air chambers and can withstand prolonged exposure to salt water. Noni is believed to have spread to Asia, Australia, and the Americas initially by seeds floating on ocean currents, and later by Polynesian traders and settlers. Noni was a founder crop of the original peoples who populated the Hawaiian Islands.

Modern research has identified several important nutritional compounds in noni. Noni fruit is full of many powerful antioxidants and compounds that support health such as selenium (skin elasticity, skin health), xeronine (cell structure health and regeneration), glycosides (defense against free radicals), scopoletin (anti-inflammatory properties), terpine (helps the body detoxify), limonene, and anthraquinones (antiseptic properties, particularly effective for people with compromised immune systems). Studies have suggested an exciting finding: that noni increases the efficacy of the immune system by stimulating white blood cells via the power of long-chain sugars (polysaccharides). Polysaccharide compounds (such as 6-D-glucopyranose penta-acetate) found in the fruit are generally believed to increase the overall killing power of white blood cells.

Noni juice is a potent antimicrobial and antifungal enzymatic beverage created during the fermentation of the noni fruit. It is generally considered to have far more health properties than any other fermented fruit products, including wine and vinegar. If you live in or visit a tropical region like Hawaii, be sure to try the noni fruit fresh. You can blend up the entire ripe fruit in coconut water, strain it, and drink it on the spot! Consuming fresh

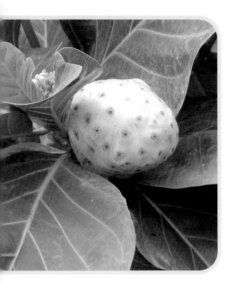

noni creates a psychoactive "high" that never seems to have any "low." It is all good news, nonstop, forever. By all indications noni appears to boost "feel-good" serotonin. Raw NoniLand™ noni powder and noni fruit leathers that contain the same psychoactive and health-enhancing properties as the fresh noni are now available.

Newly discovered compounds found in noni leaves have proven to be rich in flavonoids and other antioxidants that help protect cells and tissues from free-radical damage. Tea made from the leaves helps to improve digestion, maintain normal blood sugar levels, and eliminate toxins from the body. The tea also has antimicrobial, antibacterial, and antifungal properties. Preliminary evidence suggests that the leaves and seeds of noni contain omega-3 fatty acids.

The flavor of noni leaf tea is extremely pleasant. It tastes a bit like coca tea with hints of green tea. Noni leaf is relaxing and contains no caffeine or stimulants of any kind. No trace of the pungent odor or taste of the noni fruit or noni juice is present in the leaves of the noni tree. These leaves can be dried into noni leaf tea. Noni leaf tea is a great way to ingest the great health-giving compounds of the noni plant. Picking noni leaves from the noni tree does not damage the tree in any way; in fact, new leaves grow back swiftly and abundantly in their place.

Yacon Root: Prehistoric Prebiotic Sunflower

Yacon is a distant relative of the sunflower, with edible tubers and leaves. It is commonly grown and consumed from Colombia to northwest Argentina. Yacon is both naturally low-calorie and low in mono- and disaccharide sugars (sugars that rapidly elevate blood sugar levels). Every part of the plant has been used to help those with blood-sugar disorders.

Yacon syrup is fresh pressed from the yacon root, and has been enjoyed for centuries as a healthy, low-glycemic, natural sweetener in the Andean highlands of Peru. Yacon root can also be found in dried slices or in powdered form.

As a prebiotic, yacon is good for digestion, stimulates positive colon health, and helps with the absorption of calcium, magnesium, and B vitamins. Yacon helps to regulate friendly intestinal flora, and especially improves the growth of certain probiotics (bifidobacterium and lactobacillus species), thus helping to reduce constipation. Yacon root contains significant quantities of potassium and antioxidants. Because of its high antioxidant value, yacon is beneficial in reducing free-radical damage in the body, especially in the colon.

Fructooligosaccharides (FOS)

The root of yacon is considered the world's richest natural source of fructooligosaccharides. Most other roots and tubers store carbohydrates as starch—a polymer chain of glucose, but yacon stores carbohydrate as FOS—a polymer chain composed mainly of fructose. FOS can be considered a subgroup of inulin because it has a similar molecular structure, but with shorter fructose chains.

Standardized yacon syrup contains approximately 30 percent FOS and low proportions of simple sugars (e.g., glucose, fructose, and sucrose). The human body has no enzyme to hydrolyze FOS, so even though it tastes sweet, it passes through the digestive tract mostly unmetabolized, providing few calories. Yacon also acts as a prebiotic. The undigested portion of yacon serves as food for "friendly" bacteria (bifidobacterium and lactobacillus species), in the small intestines and colon. Clinical studies have shown that administering FOS can increase the number of these friendly bacteria in the colon while simultaneously reducing the population of harmful bacteria. Other benefits noted with FOS supplementation include increased production of beneficial short-chain fatty acids such as butyrate, increased absorption of calcium and magnesium, and improved elimination of toxic compounds. Preclinical studies indicate an increase in bone density after consumption of FOS. In addition, the beneficial effects of FOS on the presence of bifidobacterium suggest an improved absorption of vitamins such as those in the B complex.

Yacon in Blood Sugar Tests

Tests from the Universidad Nacional Mayor de San Marcos in Peru in 2004 tested how yacon syrup affects blood glucose levels. Participants (sixty nondiabetic men and women between the ages of twenty and sixty) fasted for at least eight hours before ingesting various sweeteners. Six groups were given different samples of yacon and other sweeteners. Three groups were given yacon root syrup, one group was given honey, another group was given maple syrup, and the last was given anhydrous glucose. The three groups ingesting yacon syrup had the least blood sugar variance, as measured before and after. These results showed that yacon had very little effect on glucose levels, while other sweeteners showed an immediate, significant rise and a slow decline back to normal.

Yacon helps manage cholesterol and triglyceride levels within the body, as well as fat metabolism in general. Yacon also contains glyconutrients (essential sugars or polysaccharides) and helps boost the immune system in a similar way to aloe vera. Yacon is ideal for detoxification and for low-calorie and low-sugar diets.

How to Use Yacon Products

Use yacon syrup as you would honey, agave, or maple syrup—on foods, in recipes, and to sweeten beverages with a spoonful. Yacon syrup has very little influence on the glucose tolerance curve.

Like other roots in the sunflower family (Jerusalem artichokes), yacon is extraordinarily rich in iron. In combination with other superfoods rich

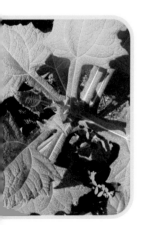

in iron, such as cacao and spirulina, one can devise an effective strategy for improving anemia and blood oxygenation.

Yacon slices can be eaten as a nonglycemic, mineral-rich snack. This is a great treat for children and a wonderful food for hikes and long-distance trips. It also keeps remarkably well.

Yacon root powder and yacon leaf powder can be added to homemade chocolates, beverages, elixirs, and desserts to support healthy blood sugar levels.

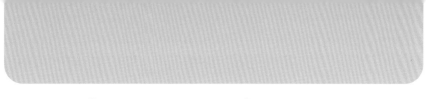

Glossary of Recipe Ingredients

Agaricus blazei—This is a medicinal mushroom originally discovered in Brazil. It is now available as a powder or capsules via the Internet or in your local health food store.

Almond milk—A "milk" made by blending raw almonds with water and then straining the mixture through a mesh bag.

Angstrom minerals—Excellent-quality liquid mineral supplements.

Blue-green algae powder—Blue-green algae is typically dried into cakes; it may then be crushed into a powder.

Burdock root—A potent wild food/herb. Burdock is exceptionally high in the mineral iron. It is one of the best blood purifiers and is the most important herb for chronic skin problems such as acne, psoriasis, and eczema. It is a great food/herb for rheumatic (inflammatory) calcification conditions, especially those associated with psoriasis. Burdock's bitter properties improve digestion and stimulate digestive juices and bile flow. Burdock is considered a diuretic, diaphoretic (increases perspiration), and a mucilaginous demulcent. The Chinese also consider burdock an aphrodisiac.

Camu Camu berry extract powder—The world's greatest vitamin C source, brought to you as a superherb powder.

Cat's Claw (uña de gato)—A popular special antiviral herb from South America.

Chanca Piedra—"The Stone Breaker." This interesting South American herb is known to help remove bad calcium and calcium-forming organisms (nanobacteria) from the body.

Chlorella powder—A green algae superfood in dried and powdered form.

Chuchuhuasi—A tree bark from the Amazon. This wonderful herb supports the lower back, reproductive system, kidneys, adrenals, and knees.

Cistanche powder—Considered a wonderful aphrodisiac in the Chinese medicine tradition. This herb is available online or at some Chinese markets.

Colloidal Gold—This extraordinary product is a beverage that helps to increase serotonin production and feelings of well-being by an unknown mechanism. It also helps protect us from stress and arthritis. This product should contain only colloidal gold and water.

Cordyceps—An extraordinary *jing* herb that helps improve the kidneys and adrenals.

Crystal Manna (blue-green algae)—AFA blue-green algae, dried in flakes.

David Wolfe's Wild Goji Berry Extract—An extract of wild Arizona goji berries made by David Wolfe and only available seasonally.

Dr. Patrick Flanagan's "Crystal Energy"—A squirt-bottle containing the mineral silicon in solution with antioxidant hydrogen and other nutrients. Squirt this in your water to improve its quality, taste, and antioxidant content.

Dried AFA—This is dried, powdered AFA blue-green algae.

Dried marine phytoplankton—A powerful, concentrated superfood powder loaded with ATP (for energy), chlorophyll (for the blood), and EPA (for the brain).

Dulse seaweed—A red-purple seaweed native to the North Atlantic. This is a favorite of raw-foodists worldwide. Dulse goes great with mashed avocadoes.

E3Live™ flakes (blue-green algae)—E3Live™ is a brand name of AFA blue-green algae. This is the product in flaked form.

E3Live™ AFA crystal flakes or dried algae flakes—E3Live™ AFA blue-green algae in light flake form.

E3Live™ fresh liquid—An E3Live™ living-liquid AFA algae product. This product is shipped to you frozen in a bottle. Thaw the product for 24 hours in your refrigerator and then consume.

Eucommia bark powder—A wonderful *jing* herb from Chinese medicine. This herb helps support the lower back, pregnancy, the skin, reproductive energy, and the kidneys.

Fluffy Citrus—A type of Sacred Heart Chocolate bar.

Gynostemma herbal tea—A wonderful Chinese herb with similar properties to ginseng, yet with a more feminine energy.

Hemp milk—This milk is made from hempseed blended with water and strained through a strainer, nut-milk bag, or fine-mesh bag.

Ho shou wu—This is a wonderful, delicious, *jing* longevity herb used in Chinese medicine. *Ho shou wu* is a root with properties that stimulate the production of "feel-good" neurotransmitters. Available as chips or as a powder.

Horsetail—A silicon-rich superherb that helps increase bone density and strength. Sometimes known as shavegrass.

Hunza raisins—A wonderful, delicious green raisin variety.

Irish moss (a.k.a. Irish sea moss)—A nutritious seaweed that turns to a gelatinous consistency when mixed with liquids and allowed to cool.

Lion's mane medicinal mushroom powders—This is the powder of the nervous system–rebuilding superherb known as Lion's Mane.

Liquid zeolites—Zeolites are cleansing minerals (based on silicon) that can be liquefied and consumed to remove heavy metals and volatile organic compounds (VOCs).

Lucuma powder—Lucuma is the "egg-fruit" of Peru. It is a delicious additive to chocolate and ice cream dishes.

Maca Extreme—A powdered form of maca extract. This product really delivers the aphrodisiac effects that maca offers. You can get more of the benefits of maca while eating less of it.

Manuka honey—A specific type of healing honey that comes from New Zealand. It possesses topical healing and stomach-rejuvenating properties.

Medicinal mushroom powders—The medicinal mushrooms are some of the most powerful herbs in the world. These mushrooms include reishi, chaga, maitake, shiitake, lion's mane, and others.

MegaHydrate™—A hydrogen and hydrating antioxidant supplement developed by Dr. Patrick Flanagan.

Mesquite powder—Mesquite is the legume-fruit of a tree native to the Americas. Native Americans have used mesquite as a nonglycemic sweetener for thousands of years. Mesquite is rich in calcium, zinc, and fiber. Mesquite powder is available online and via health food stores.

Milk thistle seed—The seed of the milk thistle plant. They are generally considered to be the best food for rejuvenating the liver.

MSM powder—Methyl-sulfonyl-methane (MSM) is a highly bioavailable form of the mineral sulfur. MSM possesses powerful rejuvenative, rejuvenating, anti-inflammatory, and healing properties.

Nama shoyu—A favorite type of soy sauce.

Nettle—A silicon- and iron-rich superherb known for its "stinging" properties when encountered in a hedge.

Non-GMO soy lecithin—This is the lecithin fraction removed from soybeans that have not been genetically modified. Lecithin is nutrition for the brain and nervous system.

NoniLand™ honey—NoniLand™ is a Hawaiian brand that supplies the best honey and noni superfood powder ever from pristine environments on the Hawaiian Islands. NoniLand™ honeys are extraordinarily rich in trace minerals and enzymes. NoniLand™ honeys range in color from clear yellows to amber red to nearly black. NoniLand™ honeys may even exceed Manuka honeys from New Zealand in healing properties.

NoniLand™ noni powder—This product consists of wild noni superfruits that are dried at low temperature and then slowly ground into a powder. This extraordinarily nutritious powder is easy to add to any lemonade, smoothie, shake, or salad dressing.

Orgono Living Silica—A joint-healing, mineralizing liquid concentrate of spring water. Orgono is highly absorbable. Its supportive qualities have been used throughout the world for more than twenty years to restore joint health, revitalize the skin, and reverse signs of aging.

Ormus Gold—This is David Wolfe's leading product. Ormus Gold is a miraculous topical healing liquid made out of pure gold and silicon. David Wolfe's Ormus Gold is the product of seventeen years of research and development. Ormus Gold is created by an alchemical process, whereby pure gold is transformed into a nonmetallic form and bound to the mineral silicon in a liquid solution. Ormus Gold was known to ancient civilizations and was said to possess magical healing properties.

Pau d'Arco—A powerful antifungal, anti-candida herb from South America. It makes a delicious tea.

Phycocyanin—The stem-cell producing, blue pigments in blue-green algae. This concentrated, powdered form of the algae is available online and in certain health food stores.

Pink salt—This is a full-spectrum rock salt that comes from a famous salt deposit in Pakistan.

Propolis tincture—An extract of bee propolis, a powerful healing substance bees produce out of sap and use to "protect their city."

Psyllium hull—The seed or seed hull of the psyllium plant. This seed gels up into a nice fiber to help move and clean digestive waste from the intestines.

Pure Radiance C® Powder—A wonderful superfood product developed by the Synergy company. It contains the extraordinary vitamin C–rich camu camu berry powder.

Pure Synergy®—A green superfood powder containing the powders of sixty superfoods, foods, and superherbs.

Purple corn extract powder—This is an antioxidant-rich, purple corn kernel extract.

Reishi—A medicinal mushroom superherb known to have extraordinary health-giving properties. This superherb is known as a super immune booster.

Rice protein—This is an excellent form of protein. It is better than soy, whey, or other forms of plant or animal protein.

Royal jelly—A special secretion the bees prepare that is fed only to the queen bee. This honey-like substance increases longevity in humans.

Sacha jergon—This is one of the great super-immunity and liver-cleansing superherbs coming out of the Amazon. Available in chips or as a superherb powder.

Sacred Chocolate™—This is the brand name of the most wonderful chocolate bar in the world (available in heart shapes).

Sprouted sunflower seeds—Raw sunflower seeds soaked in pure water for 6 to 8 hours in order to lower the enzyme inhibitors and increase the availability of nutrients.

Stevia (Vanilla Crème)—A sweetening agent and flavor that is nonglycemic and helps manage blood sugar levels.

Suma powder—This powdered root is one of the leading adaptogenic superherbs coming out of Brazil.

Sun Warrior™ *barley*—A brand of powdered barley product that contains beta-glucans for long-term energy.

Sun Warrior™ *protein powder*—This is a rice protein brand.

Super deer antler—Deer antler velvet is a hormone-building superherb from Chinese medicine. Please procure ethically harvested deer antler (the deer antler velvet can be acquired without killing or maiming the deer). Super deer antler is a liquid alcohol extract of deer antler velvet.

Super ionic minerals—A liquid mineral supplement containing ionic trace minerals.

Tocotrienols—Mechanically powdered rice bran. This is an extraordinary source of the vitamin E varieties known as tocotrienols.

Vita-Mix®—A high-speed blender brand. This is a recommended appliance for any superfood kitchen.

Wild jungle peanuts—A variety of original, beautiful, aflatoxin-free peanuts from Ecuador.

Yacon syrup—A syrup made out of the root of the giant sunflower plant indigenous to Peru.

Zeolites—A type of "super clay" that sponges up toxins such as heavy metals and volatile organic compounds from the body. Available as a powder or in liquid form.

Appendix I
Nutritional Information

Goji Berry

Minerals

Goji contains 21 trace minerals including:

Calcium

Copper

Geranium (anti-cancer mineral rarely found in foods)

Iron (11mg/100g)

Magnesium

Phosphorus

Selenium

Zinc

Vitamins

Vitamin A (super-antioxidant, improves eye and nerve health)

Vitamin C (73mg/100g)

Vitamin B-complex (helps convert food into energy, increases energy, improves mood)

B1

B2

B6

Vitamin E (rarely found in fruits)

Amino Acids (Protein)

Contains 18 amino acids (of which eight are essential for life)

50 percent are free-form amino acids

More protein than whole wheat (13%)

A complete protein source

Analysis Test	Methods	Results
Energy	Atwater Method, USDA Handbook 74	391 Calories/100g
Calories from Fat	Atwater Method, USDA Handbook 74	74 Calories/100g
Protein (N X 6.25)	AOAC 990.03	11.70%
Fat	AOAC 990.03	8.20%
Saturated Fats	AOAC 991.39	2.80%
Monounsaturated Fats	AOAC 991.39	1.10%
Polyunsaturated Fats	AOAC 991.39	4.30%
Beta-carotene	AOAC 970.64	28,7000IU/100g
Cholesterol	JAOCS Vol 76 No 4, pg 902-906	1mg/100g

(continued on next page)

Analysis Test	Methods	Results
Carbohydrates	Atwater Method, USDA Handbook 74	67.70%
Total Sugars	AOAC 971.18	57.40%
Total Dietary Fiber	AOAC 991.43	10.00%
Sodium (Na)	AOAC 968.08	294 mg/100g
Vitamin A	J Sci Fd Agri, Vol 29 Pg767-722	10IU/100g
Retinol Equivalents	J Sci Fd Agri, Vol 29 Pg767-722	1,610 RE/100g
Vitamin C	AOAC 967.21	<1mg/100g
Calcium (Ca)	AOAC 968.08	60.0 mg/100g
Iron (Fe)	AOAC 968.08	6.9 mg/100g
Total Polysaccharides	Calculated	30%

Amino Acid	Free Amino Acid	Water Soluble Amino Acid	Total
Aspartic Acid	1.21	0.4	1.76
Threonine	0.07	0.07	0.29
Serine	0.14	0.11	0.43
Glutamic acid	0.63	0.28	1.27
Glycine	0.04	0.03	0.19
Alanine	0.37	0.18	0.64
Valine	0.05	0.05	0.26
Methionine	0.00	0.00	0.04
Isoleucine	0.04	0.04	0.2
Leucine	0.09	0.03	0.3
Tyrosine	0.05	0.00	0.16
Phenylalanine	0.06	0.02	0.16
Lysine	0.02	0.02	0.16
Ammonia	0.3	0.07	0.58
Histidine	0.04	0.02	0.1
Arginine	0.19	0.09	0.45
Proline	0.65	0.13	0.91
TOTAL AMOUNT:	3.95	1.54	7.9
TOTAL %:	50	19	100

Amino Acid	Amount mg/100mg
Aspartic Acid	1.55 mg/100mg
Threonine	0.37 mg/100mg
Serine	0.47 mg/100mg
Glutamic acid	1.23 mg/100mg
Glycine	1.23 mg/100mg
Alanine	0.43 mg/100mg
Cystine	0.11 mg/100mg
Valine	0.37 mg/100mg
Methionine	0.10 mg/100mg
Isoleucine	0.29 mg/100mg
Leucine	0.45 mg/100mg
Tyrosine	0.15 mg/100mg
Phenylalanine	0.26 mg/100mg
Lysine	0.31 mg/100mg
Ammonia	0.38 mg/100mg
Histidine	0.15 mg/100mg
Arginine	0.94 mg/100mg
Tryptophan	0.10 mg/100mg
Proline	1.08 mg/100mg
TOTAL:	9.14 mg/100mg

Polysaccharides and Their Properties

Very large, long-chain sugar molecules that are nourishment for macrophages (large white blood cells) in the gut wall. The macrophages are then transported to other immune cells, setting off a chain of defensive events in the human body.

Immune stimulant
Inhibits tumor growth
Anti-cancer
Neutralizes side effects of chemo-
   therapy and radiation
Normalizes blood pressure
Balances blood sugar
Combats autoimmune disease
Anti-inflammatory
Balances immune function
Increases calcium absorption
Lowers cholesterol and blood lipids
Normalize cell growth
Restore and repair DNA
Scavenge free oxygen radicals

Lycium Barbarum Polysaccharides (LBP 1–4)

glycoconjugates (essential
   cell sugars)
rhamnose
xylose
glucose
mannose
arabinose
galactose

Antioxidants

ORAC (Oxygen Radical Absorbance Capacity) 133 per gram
(Antioxidant measurement)

Vitamin C	Super antioxidant
Beta-carotene	Immunity
Cystine	Immunity and healthy stomach lining
B2 (riboflavin)	Conversion of carbohydrates into fuel
Manganese	Healthy blood, bone, cartilage
Zinc	Wound healing, fertility, vision, immunity
Copper	Energy, hormonal function, healthy skin
Selenium	Healthy liver, thyroid, immunity, cancer protection

Carotenoids

Increases longevity
Beta-carotene (goji is one of the richest known sources)
26,000 and 8,000 IU/100g

Tetraterpenoids

Zeaxanthin (protects vision)
Physalin

Other Active Naturally Occurring Ingredients

Beta-Sitosterol

Anti-inflammatory
Lowers cholesterol
Treats sexual impotence
Treats prostate enlargement

Betaine (0.1%)

Protects DNA
Increases choline production by liver
Calms nervousness
Enhances memory
Promotes muscle growth
Protection against fatty liver disease
Aids in liver detoxification

Essential fatty acids

Produces hormones
Assists brain and nervous system function
Linoleic acid

Flavonoids

Antioxidant
Protect cell membranes

Solavetivone

Antifungal
Antibacterial

Physalin

Anti-cancer
Anti-leukemia
Immune system booster
Fights leukemia
Used in hepatitis B treatment

Sesquiterpenoids

Stimulates the glandular production of Humane Growth Hormone
Increase longevity
Cyperone (a sesquiterpene)
Used in the treatment of cervical cancer
Benefits heart and blood pressure
Relieves menstrual discomfort
Has been used with treatment of cervical cancer
Solavetivone

Tetraterpenoids

Zeaxanthin
Physalin

Sources

Mindell, Earl, and Rick Handel. *Goji: the Himalayan Health Secret.* Texas: Momentum Media, 2003.

Teeguarden, R. *The Ancient Wisdom of the Chinese Tonic Herbs.* New York: Warner Books, Inc., 1998.

Gross, P.M., X. Zhang, and R. Zhang. *Wolfberry: Nature's Bounty of Nutrition and Health.* Booksurge Publishing, 2006.

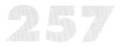

Cacao

Analytical Report (Cacao Nibs www.sacredchocolate.com)

All results are reflected per 100 grams

Protein	15.4 grams
Carbohydrate (Total)	29.4 grams
Fat (Total)	48.0 grams
Moisture	3.9 grams
Ash	3.3 grams
Calories	611
Calories from Fat	432
Saturated Fat	27.6 grams
Trans Fat	0.25 grams
Dietary Fiber	22.3 grams
Sugars	0.1 grams
Sodium	53 mg
Calcium	58 mg
Iron	202 mg
Magnesium	342 mg
Vitamin A	20 (IU)
Vitamin C	44 mg

*Northeast Laboratories, Inc.; Cacao Nibs, Analytical Report

The Cacao Bean's Natural Chemical Constituents and Their Concentrations (when available)

Acetic acid 1,520–7,100 ppm
Alanine 10,400 ppm
Amylase
Anandamide
Arabinose
Arginine 800+ ppm
Ascorbic acid 31 ppm
Aspariginase
Beta Theosterol
Caffeic acid
Caffeine, Petiole 51–525 ppm or 500–12,900 ppm, Skin 130–723 ppm
Calcium 800–1,100 ppm
Camposterol
Carbohydrates 347,000–445,000 ppm
Catalase
Catechins 30,000–35,000 ppm
Chloride 120 ppm
Chromium (10 times more than whole wheat, highest of any major food)
Citric acid 4,500–7,500 ppm
Copper 24 ppm
Coumarin
Cyanidin-glycoside 4,000–5,000 ppm
Dopamine
Epigallocatechin
Ergosterol
Fat 371,000–582,300 ppm
Fiber 59,000–89,000 ppm
Glucose 3,000 ppm
Glutamic acid 10,200 ppm
Glycine 900 ppm
Histamine
Histidine 800 ppm
Iron 36–37 ppm
Iron oxide 40 ppm
Isoleucine 5,600 ppm
L-epicatechin 27,000 ppm
Lactic acid
Leucine
Leucocyanidins 14,000–35,000 ppm
Linalol 5 ppm
Linoleic acid
Linolenic acid
Lipase
Lysine 800 ppm
Lysophosphatidylcholine
Magnesium
Mannose
N-linoleoylethanolamine— Anandamide reuptake inhibitor

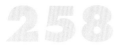

N-oleolethanolamine—Ananda-
mide reuptake inhibitor
Niacin 17–18 ppm
Nicotinamide 21 ppm
Nitrogen 22,800 ppm
Oleic acid 190,000–217,000 ppm
Oleo-Dipalmatin 76,500–92,800
ppm
Oxalic acid 1,520–5,000 ppm
Palmitic acid
Pantothenic acid (Vitamin B5) 13
ppm
Pectin
Pentose
Peroxidase
Phenylacetic acid
Phenylalanine 5,600 ppm
Phenylethylamine
Phosphatidyl-choline 92–1,328
ppm
Phospholipids
Phosphorus 3,600–5,571 ppm
Polyphenols 78,000–100,000 ppm
Proline 7,200 ppm
Protein 120,000–180,000 ppm
Purine 30,000–40,000 ppm
Pyridoxine (Vitamin B6) 1 ppm
Riboflavin (Vitamin B2) 1–4 ppm
Serine 8,800 ppm
Serotonin
Sitosterol
Starch 60,000 ppm
Stearic acid
Tannins 75,400 ppm
Theobromine 10,000–33,500 ppm
Theophylline 3,254–4,739 ppm—
Theophylline is a methyl-
xanthine with diuretic and
bronchial smooth muscle
relaxant properties.
Thiamine (Vitamin B1) 1–3 ppm
Threonine 1,400 ppm

Tocopherol (beta, gamma,
Vitamin E)
Tryptophan
Tyramine
Tyrosine 5,700 ppm
Valine 5,700 ppm
Vanillic acid
Water 36,000 ppm
Xylose

Sources

www.sacredchocolate.com
Wolfe, David, and Shazzie. *Naked Chocolate.* Berkeley: North Atlantic Books,
2005.
Dr. Duke's Phytochemical and Ethnobotanical Databases

Maca

Minerals

Calcium (higher than potatoes)
(350–500mg/100g)
Copper
Iron (higher than potatoes)
Magnesium
Phosphorus (300–350mg/100g)
Potassium (1600–2000mg/100g)
Iodine
Zinc
Sulfur
Iron
Sodium
Manganese
Aluminum
Tin

Vitamins

Vitamin B1 (thiamine)
Vitamin B2 (riboflavin)
Vitamin C
Vitamin E

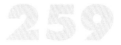

Amino Acids
Alanine
Arginine
Aspartic acid
Glutamine
Glycine
Histidine
OH-proline
Isoleucine
Leucine
Lysine
Methionine
Phenylalanine
Proline
Sarcosine
Serine
Threonine
Tyrosine
Valine

More Nutrients and Facts
Carbohydrates   59%
Protein   10.2%
Fiber   8.5%
Lipids   2.2%
Sterols
  Brassicasterol
  Erogosterol
  Ergostadienol
  Campesterol
  Sitosterol
  Stigmasterol
Fatty Acids
  Oleic
  Lauric
  Myristic
  Palmitic
  Palmitoleic
  Linoleic
  Arachidic
  Steric
  Behanic
  Nervonic

Lignoceric
Tridecanoic
7-tridecanoic
Perntadecanoic
7-pentadecanoic
Heptadecanoic
9-heptadecanoic
Nonadecanoic
11-nonadecanoic
15-eicosenoic
Alkaloids
  Macaina 1-4 (Chacón)
  Macamides
  Macaenes (Zheng)
Glucosinolates (anti-cancer,
  antimutagenic, anticarcinogenic)
Indole3-carbinol
Isothiocyanates
P-methoxybenzyl isothi ocyanate
  (aphrodisiac properties)

Sources

Ley, B.M. *MACA: Adaptogen and Hormonal Regulator.* Minnesota: BL Publications, 2003.

Bee Products

Bee Pollen

Minerals
Calcium
Phosphorus
Potassium
Iron
Copper
Iodine
Zinc
Sulfur
Sodium
Chlorine
Magnesium
Manganese
Molybdenum

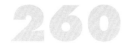

Selenium
Boron
Silica
Titanium

Vitamins

Provitamin A
B-1 Thiamin
B-2 Riboflavin
B-3 Niacin
B-5
B-6 Pyridoxine
B-12 (cyanocobalamin)
Pantothenic Acid
Vitamin C
Vitamin F
Vitamin D
Vitamin E
Vitamin H
Vitamin K
Vitamin P
Folic Acid
Choline
Inositol
Rutin

Other Nutrients

Amino acids
Carbohydrates
Fatty acids
Enzymes and coenzymes
Fats

Honey

Average Composition of Honey
(all values % except for pH)

Component	Average	Range
Moisture	17.2%	12.2–22.9%
Fructose	38.4	30.9–44.3
Glucose	30.3	22.9–40.7
Sucrose	1.3	0.2–7.6
Maltose	7.3	2.7–16.0
Higher Sugars	1.4	0.1–3.8
Acid as Gluconic	0.57	0.17–1.17
Ash	0.169	0.02–1.03
Nitrogen	0.041	0.00–0.13
pH	3.91	3.42–6.10

Sources

Kacera, Walter "Shantree." *Pollen Power: Nectar of Life.* Ayurvedic Nutritionist and Herbalist, 2002.

Royal Jelly

Analysis of royal jelly reveals all major vitamins: A, B-complex, C, D, and E. It contains a natural antibiotic—decanoic acid—sulfur, and over 5% fatty acids, 12% protein, and nearly 3% "unidentifiable" substances. The moisture content is 66%. Natural hormones, essential sugars, nucleic acids, vegetable gelatin, gamma globulin, and other fascinating nutrients are also found in royal jelly.

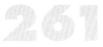
Propolis

Like all beehive products, propolis is made of locally gathered substances of plant origin. Propolis differs in composition from place to place. It typically consists of:

30% beeswax
55% resins
10% aromatic ethers and essential oils
5% pollen.

A sampling of chemical ingredients often includes:

B vitamins	ferulic acid
caffeic acid	iron
calcium	manganese
chrysin	silicon
cinnamic acid	tectochrysin
cinnamyl alcohol	vanadium
copper	vanillan
E vitamins	vitamin C

Propolis may contain up to 27 additional compounds that are not clearly scientifically understood in their composition and/or effects.

Spirulina

Essential Minerals and Trace Elements

Mineral	Amount
Potassium	15,400 mg/kg
Calcium	1,315 mg/kg
Zinc	39 mg/kg
Magnesium	1,915 mg/kg
Manganese	25 mg/kg
Selenium	0.40 ppm
Iron	580 mg/kg
Phosphorus	8,942 mg/kg

Minerals (per 10 grams)

Mineral	Amount
Calcium	12 mg
Magnesium	14.4 mg
Iron	3.18 mg
Phosphorus	31.2 mg
Potassium	45.6 mg
Sodium	21.9 mg
Manganese	78 mcg
Zinc	36 mcg
Boron	30 mcg
Copper	3 mcg
Molybdenum	3 mcg

Vitamins (per 10 grams)

Vitamin	Amount
Beta-carotene	10 mg
Vitamin A (100% as Beta-carotene)	15,030 IU
Vitamin B1 (Thiamin)	102 mcg
Vitamin B2 (Riboflavin)	99 mcg
Vitamin B3 (Niacin)	621 mcg
Vitamin B6	13 mcg
Vitamin B12	6.6 mcg
Inositol	2.04 mg
Biotin	0.969 mg
Folic Acid	0.9 mcg
Pantothenic	12 mcg
Pyridoxine (B6)	3 mg/kg
Biotin	0.4 mg/kg
Cobalamin (B12)	2 mg/kg
Pantothenic Acid	11 mg/kg
Folic Acid	0.5 mg/kg
Inositol	350 mg/kg
Niacin	118 mg/kg
Riboflavin (B2)	40 mg/kg
Thiamine (B1)	55 mg/kg
Tocopherol (Vit E)	190 mg/kg

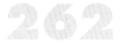

Amino Acids
Eight Essential Amino Acids

Amino Acid	%
Isoleucine	4.13%
Leucine	5.80%
Lysine	4.00%
Methionine	2.17%
Phenylalanine	3.95%
Threonine	4.17%
Tryptophan	1.13%
Valine	6.00%

Non-essential Amino Acids

Amino Acid	%
Alanine	5.82%
Arginine	5.98%
Aspartic Acid	6.34%
Cystine	0.67%
Glutamic Acid	8.94%
Glycine	3.50%
Histidine	1.08%
Proline	2.97%
Serine	4.00%
Tyrosine	4.60%

Overall Composition of Spirulina
Chemical Analysis of Spirulina

Protein	71%
Crude Fiber	0.90%
Carbohydrates	16.90%
Fat	7.00%
Cholesterol (less than)	0.05%
Moisture	7.00%

General Composition Analysis of Another Spirulina

Protein	60%
Carbohydrates	19%
Lipids	6%
Minerals	8%
Moisture	7%

Vitamin Analysis of Spirulina (average)

Biotin	0.4 mg/kg
Vitamin B12	2 mg/kg
D-Ca-Pantothenate	11 mg/kg
Folic Acid	0.5 mg/kg
Inositol	350 mg/kg
Nicotinic Acid	118 mg/kg
Vitamin B6	3 mg/kg
Vitamin B2	40 mg/kg
Vitamin B1	55 mg/kg
Vitamin E	190 mg/kg

Mineral Analysis of Spirulina (average)

Calcium	1,315 mg/kg
Phosphorus	8,942 mg/kg
Iron	580 mg/kg
Sodium	412 mg/kg
Magnesium	1,915 mg/kg
Manganese	25 mg/kg
Zinc	39 mg/kg
Potassium	15,400 mg/kg
Selenium	0.4 mg/kg

Other Components (average)

Nucleic Acids	4.50%
Carotenoids	0.40%
Chlorophyll	0.80%
Crude Protein	71%

Essential Amino Acids

Isoleucine	4.10%
Leucine	5.80%
Lysine	4.00%
Methionone	2.20%
Phenylalanine	4.00%
Threonine	4.20%
Tryptophan	1.10%
Valine	6.00%

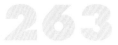
Non-Essential Amino Acids

Alanine	5.80%
Arginine	6.00%
Aspartic Acid	6.40%
Cystine	0.70%
Glutamic Acid	8.90%
Glycine	3.50%
Histidine	1.10%
Proline	3.00%
Serine	4.00%
Tyrosine	4.60%

Polysaccharides and Phytonutrients per 10 grams (% spirulina)

Gamma-Linolenic Acid (GLA)	130 mg	1.3%
Glycolipids (Lipid)	200 mg	2.0%
Sulfolipids (Glycolipids)	10 mg	0.1%
Polysaccharides	460 mg	4.6%

Antioxidants per 10 grams

Beta-carotene 9-cis	1.60 mg
Beta-carotene 13-cis	0.52 mg
Beta-carotene 15-cis	0.12 mg
Beta-carotene all-trans	7.80 mg
Zeaxanthin	0.95 mg
Chlorophyll	23.70 mg
Total carotenoids*	14 mg
Phycocyanin	333 mg
Superoxide Dismutase**	2,640 units

*Includes alpha carotene, beta cryptoxanthin, and others.

**Reported as units Ferric S.O.D.

Carotenoid Profile

Carotenoid	**Amount**
Alpha-carotene	traces
Beta-carotene	1,700 mg/kg
Xanthophylls	1,000 mg/kg
Cryptoxanthin	556 mg/kg
Echinenone	439 mg/kg
Zeaxanthin	316 mg/kg
Lutein	289 mg/kg

Other Active Naturally Occurring Ingredients (per 10 grams)

Omega-6 Family

Gamma-Linolenic (GLA)	30 mg
Essential Linoleic	33 mg
Dihomogamma Linolenic	1.59 mg

Omega-3 Family

Alpha-Linolenic	0.0435 mg
Docosahexaenoic (DHA)	0.0435 mg

Monoenoic Family

Palmitoleic	5.94 mg
Oleic	0.51 mg
Erucic	0.072 mg

Sources

Challem, Jack J. *Spirulina.* New Canaan, CT: Keats Publishing, 1981.

McCauley, B. *Confessions of a Body Builder.* Lansing, MI: Spartan Enterprises, 2000.

http://www.mallorcaspirit.com/Alternative_Medicine_directory/spirulina.html

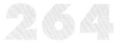

Blue-Green Algae

Minerals

Boron	0.05 mg
Calcium	4.86 mg
Chloride	0.02 mg
Chromium	0.18 mcg
Cobalt	0.69 mcg
Copper	1.49 mcg
Fluoride	13.21 mcg
Germanium	0.09 mcg
Iodine	18 mcg
Iron	121.69 mcg
Magnesium	0.76 mg
Manganese	11.12 mcg
Molybdenum	1.15 mcg
Nickel	1.84 mcg
Potassium	4.16 mcg
Phosphorus	1.82 mcg
Selenium	0.23 mcg
Silicon	65.2 mcg
Sodium	0.94 mg
Tin	0.172 mcg
Titanium	16.17 mcg
Vanadium	0.96 mcg
Zinc	6.51 mcg

Minerals (per gram)

Boron	14.0 mcg
Calcium	12.70 mg
Chloride	0.47 mg
Chromium	0.53 mcg
Cobalt	2.00 mcg
Copper	4.30 mcg
Fluoride	38.00 mcg
Germanium	0.27 mcg
Iodine	0.53 mcg
Iron	0.37 mg
Magnesium	2.20 mg
Manganese	32.0 mcg
Molybdenum	3.30 mcg
Nickel	5.3 mcg
Phosphorus	5.20 mg
Potassium	12.00 mcg

Selenium	0.67 mcg
Silicon	186.70 mcg
Sodium	2.70 mg
Tin	0.47 mcg
Titanium	23.3 mcg
Vanadium	2.70 mcg
Zinc	18.70 mcg

Vitamins

Provitamin A Beta-carotene	1890 IU
Thiamin (B1)	27 mcg
Riboflavin (B2)	49 mcg
Niacin (B3)	0.05 mg
Pantothenic Acid (B5)	2.38 mcg
Pyridoxine (B6)	3.85 mcg
Inositol	55.50 mcg
Vitamin E	0.59 IU
Ascorbic Acid (Vitamin C)	2.34 mcg
Biotin	0.10 mcg
Folic Acid	0.73 mcg
Choline	0.80 mcg
Cobalamin (B12)	2.80 mcg
Vitamin K	34 mcg

Vitamins (AFA Algae)

Vitamin B1 (thiamine)
Vitamin B2 (riboflavin)
Vitamin B3 (niacin)
Pantothenic acid (B5)
Vitamin B6 (pyridoxine)
Folic Acid (B9)
Vitamin B12
Vitamin C (ascorbic acid)
Choline
Biotin
Vitamin E

Appendix I

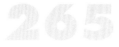

Amino Acids (AFA Algae)
Typical Amino Acid Content (per 15ml)

Essential Amino Acids

Arginine	13.19 mg
Histidine	3.12 mg
Isoleucine	10.06 mg
Leucine	18.04 mg
Lysine	12.15 mg
Methionine	2.43 mg
Phenylalanine	8.68 mg
Threonine	11.52 mg
Tryptophan	2.42 mg
Valine	11.10 mg

Non-essential Amino Acids

Alanine	16.30 mg
Asparagine	15.91 mg
Aspartic Acid	2.43 mg
Cystine	0.69 mg
Glutamic Acid	1.39 mg
Glutamine	27.06 mg
Glycine	10.06 mg
Proline	10.13 mg
Serine	10.01 mg
Tyrosine	5.89 mg

Essential	Semi-Essential	Non-Essential
Isoleucine	Arginine	Alanine
Leucine	Histidine	Aspartic Acid
Lysine		Cystine
Methionine		Glutamic Acid
Tryptophan		Proline
Threonine		Serine
Phenylalanine		Tyrosine
Valine		

Polysaccharides
Other Occurring Nutrients

Essential Fatty Acids

Alpha-Linolenic Acid (Omega 3)
10.70 mg
Gamma-Linolenic Acid (Omega 6)
2.15 mg

Typical Nutrient Composition (15ml)

Protein	< 1 gram
Fat	< 1 gram
Carbohydrate	< 1 gram
Fiber	1.50%
Moisture	94 to 95%
Chlorophyll	0.59%
Calories	3.9 Cal/0.016 kJ

Antioxidants
Beta-carotene

1–2% Chlorophyll
Helps the body obtain more oxygen
Aids digestion
Anti-inflammatory
Fights gum disease
Prevents infection
Minimizing the effects of pollution
Accelerates wound healing
Internal deodorizer
Combats bad breath and body odor
Stimulates regeneration of damaged liver cells
Increases circulation
Balances alkalinity
Aids in transmission of nerve impulses that control contraction in the heart
Strong cleansing and detoxification
15% Phycocyanin (blue pigments that increase stem cell production)
Lipids (omega-3 fatty acids that protect the nervous system)

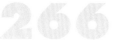
Complex carbohydrates (polysaccharides that support long-term energy and improve the immune system).

Sources

McKeith, Gillian. *Miracle Superfood: Wild Blue-Green Algae.* Los Angeles: Keats Publishing, 1999.

Earth's Essential Elements E3Live,™ *DATA SHEET Klamath Lake Blue-Green Algae.* Klamath Falls, OR: Vision, Inc., n.d.

Marine Phytoplankton

Minerals

Elements	Result
Boron	2.843 mcg/75mg
Calcium	142.500 mcg/75mg
Chromium	0.014 mcg/75mg
Copper	0.384 mcg/75mg
Iodine	1.210 mcg/75mg
Iron	90.000 mcg/75mg
Magnesium	286.500 mcg/75mg
Manganese	19.800 mcg/75mg
Molybdenum	0.023 mcg/75mg
Phosphorus	960.000 mcg/75mg
Potassium	975.000 mcg/75mg
Selenium	<0.010 mcg/75mg
Sodium	682.500 mcg/75mg
Sulfur	504.000 mcg/75mg
Vanadium	<0.069 mcg/75mg
Zinc	1.673 mcg/75mg

Vitamins

Folic Acid	0.053 mcg/75mg
Vitamin A	30.00 mcg/75mg
Vitamin B1 (Thiamine)	1.300 mcg/75mg
Vitamin B2 (Riboflavin)	7.000 mcg/75mg
Vitamin B3 (Niacin)	11.00 mcg/75mg
Vitamin B5 (Pantothenic acid)	8.000 mcg/75mg
Vitamin B6 (Pyridoxine)	0.990 mcg/75mg

Amino Acids

Isoleucine	1.275 mg/75mg
Leucine	2.625 mg/75mg
Lysine	2.175 mg/75mg
Methionine	0.825 mg/75mg
Phenylalanine	1.350 mg/75mg
Proline	2.925 mg/75mg
Threonine	1.725 mg/75mg
Tryptophan	0.600 mg/75mg
Valine	1.800 mg/75mg
Alanine	2.325 mg/75mg
Arginine	2.325 mg/75mg
Aspartic Acid	3.225 mg/75mg
Glutamic Acid	4.650 mg/75mg
Glycine	1.800 mg/75mg
Histidine	0.600 mg/75mg
Tyrosine	1.050 mg/75mg

General Composition of a Liquid Marine Phytoplankton Product

Marine Phytoplankton (*Nannochloropsis*) preserved in ocean-derived mineral concentrate
(Serving Size = 0.2 tsp), Ionic Trace Mineral Solution
Serving Size = 1.52 gm

Appendix I

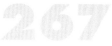

Assay	Content/100 gm	Per Serving
Saturated Fat	.230gm calculated as acids	0.0035 gm
Sum of Fatty Acids	1.18 gm calculated as triglycerides	0.018 gm
Vitamin B12	3.76 mcg	0.057 mcg
Lecithin Phospholipids by HPLC-ELSD		
Phosphatidic Acid (PA)	< 0.50 gm	
Phosphatidylethanolamine (PE)	< 0.80 gm	
Phosphatidylcholine (PC)	< 0.70 gm	
Phosphatidylserine (PS)	< 0.40 gm	
Phosphatidylinositol (PI)	< 0.50 gm	
Lyso Phosphatidylcholine (LPC)	< 0.50 gm	
Orac-Hydrophilic (MLS)	3.81 te	
Orac-Lipophilic	0.058 te	
Lipophilic	0.464 umol te/ml	
Total ORAC	4.27 umol te/ml	
Vitamin D by HPLC	112 IU	1.71 IU
	As Vitamin D3	
	< 20.0 IU	< 0.305 IU
	As Vitamin D2	
Conjugated Linoleic Acid	< 0.005 gm	
	Calculated as triglycerides	

Fatty Acids

	Content/100 gm	Per Serving
4:0 Butyric	< 0.005 gm	
6:0 Caproic	< 0.005 gm	
8:0 Caprylic	< 0.005 gm	
10:0 Capric	< 0.005 gm	
12:0 Lauric	0.007 gm	0.0001 gm
14:0 Myristic	0.011 gm	0.00017 gm
14:1 Myristoleic	< 0.005 gm	
15:0 Pentadecanoic	< 0.005 gm	
15:1 Pentadecenoic	< 0.005 gm	
16:0 Palmitic	0.202 gm	0.00307 gm
16:1 Palmitoleic	0.025 gm	0.00038 gm
17:0 Heptadecanoic	< 0.005 gm	
17:1 Heptadecenoic	< 0.005 gm	
18:0 Stearic	0.011 gm	0.00017 gm
4:0 Butyric	< 0.005 gm	
6:0 Caproic	< 0.005 gm	
8:0 Caprylic	< 0.005 gm	
10:0 Capric	< 0.005 gm	

Assay	Content/100 gm	Per Serving
12:0 Lauric	0.007 gm	0.0001 gm
14:0 Myristic	0.011 gm	0.00017 gm
14:1 Myristoleic	< 0.005 gm	
15:0 Pentadecanoic	< 0.005 gm	
15:1 Pentadecenoic	< 0.005 gm	
16:0 Palmitic	0.202 gm	0.00307 gm
16:1 Palmitoleic	0.025 gm	0.00038 gm
17:0 Heptadecanoic	< 0.005 gm	
17:1 Heptadecenoic	< 0.005 gm	
18:0 Stearic	0.011 gm	0.00017 gm
18:1 Trans (total including Elaidic)	< 0.005 gm	
18:1 Oleic	0.201 gm	0.00306 gm
18:2 Trans (total including Linolaidic)	< 0.005 gm	
18:2 Linoleic	0.467 gm	0.00710 gm
20:0 Arachidic	< 0.005 gm	
18:3 Gamma-Linolenic (GLA)	< 0.005 gm	
20:1 Eicosenoic	< 0.005 gm	
18:3 Linolenic (ALA)	0.228 gm	0.00347 gm
18:4 Octadecatetraenoic	< 0.005 gm	
20:2 Eicosadienoic	< 0.005 gm	
22:0 Behenic	< 0.005 gm	
22:1 Erucic	< 0.005 gm	
20:3 Eicosatrienoic	< 0.005 gm	
20:4 Arachidonic (ARA)	< 0.005 gm	
20:5 Eicosapentaenoic (EPA)	0.014 gm	0.00021 gm
24:0 Lignoceric	0.011 gm	0.00017 gm
22:5 Docosapentaenoic (DPA)	< 0.005 gm	
22:6 Docosahexaenoic (DHA)	< 0.005 gm	
Omega-3	0.242 gm, calculated as triglycerides	0.00368 gm
Omega-6	0.467 gm, calculated as triglycerides	0.00710 gm
Total Trans-fatty Acids	< 0.005 gm, calculated as acids	
Monounsaturated Fat	0.216 gm, calculated as acids	0.00328 gm
Polyunsaturated Fat	0.678 gm, calculated as acids	0.0103 gm

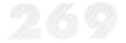
More Composition Info on Gesundheit Marine Phytoplankton (dried)

Nutritional Proxy Test

Parameter	Result
Protein	47.50%
Ash	7.20%
Energy	422 Cal/ 100 gm
Energy	1765 KJ/ 100 gm
Carbohydrates	29.40%
Fat	12.70%
Moisture	3.20%
Crude Fiber	0.10%

Fatty Acid Profile

EPA 9.3 mg/gm
DHA 4.9 mg/gm
Omega-6 Fatty Acid (Linoleic Acid)
   3.4 mg/gm
Gamma-Linolenic 3.4 mg/gm
Beta-carotene (by HPLC) *
Vitamin C (by HPLC) **
Iodine (as per USP) ***

Note:
*A number of carotenoids were found to be present in the sample. It could be Xanthophyll or other types of carotenoids.
**Vitamin C is present but could not be quantified.
***Iodine is present but could not be quantified.

Macro Nutrients

Carbohydrates	27.00 mg/75mg
Lipids	2.445 mg/75mg
Proteins	36.375 mg/75mg
Ash	6.600 mg/75mg
Moisture	3.490 mg/75mg
Nitrogen	5.820 mg/75mg
Calories	3.670 Kcal/g
Total Pigments	23.300 mcg/75mg

Aloe Vera Leaf

Minerals

In parts per million (ppm) when available

Calcium	4,600
Chlorine	
Chromium	
Cobalt	
Copper	
Germanium	
Iron	300
Magnesium	930
Manganese	0.6
Phosphorus	940
Potassium	850
Selenium	2.3
Silicon	2.2
Sodium	510
Sulfur	
Tin	11
Zinc	770

Vitamins

In parts per million (ppm) when available

Vitamin B1: Thiamin	0.8
Vitamin B2: Riboflavin	
Vitamin B3: Niacin	64
Vitamin B9: Folic Acid	200
Vitamin C	6,260
Vitamin E	
Choline	

Amino Acids and Amino Acid Groups

In parts per million (ppm) when available

Alanine	15,769
Arginine	78,216
Asparagine	
Aspartic Acid	
Creatinine	15
Glutamic Acid	43,256

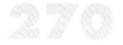

Glutamine	20,670
Glycine	5,030
Histidine	2,327
Isoleucine	8,526
Leucine	6,952
Lysine	7,748
Phenylalanine	7,103
Proline	3,339
Serine	23,540
Threonine	14,652
Tyrosine	5,073
Valine	12,769

Sugars and Polysaccharides

In parts per million (ppm) when available

Arabinose	
Fructose	
Glucose	1,030
Galactose	100
Mannose	
Rhamnose	
Xylose	

Antioxidants

In parts per million (ppm) when available

Beta-carotene	3

Enzymes

In parts per million (ppm) when available

Amylase	20
Catalase	
Lipase	16

Other Biologically Active Components

In parts per million (ppm) when available

Anthraquinones	300,000
Aloins	300,000
Purine	56

Sources

Dr. Duke's Phytochemical and Ethnobotanical Databases
http://sun.ars-grin.gov:8080/npgspub/xsql/duke/plantdisp.xsql?taxon=58

Hempseed

Minerals

Phosphorus	36.46%
Calcium	23.64%
Potassium	20.28%
Silica	11.90%
Magnesium	5.70%
Iron	1.00%
Sodium	0.78%
Sulfur	0.19%
Chlorine	0.08%

Vitamins

Vitamin E	30 mg/g
Vitamin C	14 mg/g
Vitamin B1	9 mg/g
Vitamin B2	11 mg/g
Vitamin B3	25 mg/g
Vitamin B6	3 mg/g

Amino Acids (Whole Hempseed)

(mg/g hempseed)

Alanine	9.6 mg/g
Arginine	18.8 mg/g
Aspartic Acid (and asparagine)	19.8 mg/g
Cystine (and cysteine)	1.2 mg/g
Glutamic Acid (and glutamine)	34.8 mg/g
Glycine	9.7 mg/g
Histidine	2.5 mg/g
Isoleucine	1.5 mg/g
Leucine	7.1 mg/g
Lysine	4.3 mg/g

Methionine	2.6 mg/g
Phenylalanine	3.5 mg/g
Proline	7.3 mg/g
Serine	8.6 mg/g
Threonine	3.7 mg/g
Tryptophan	0.6 mg/g
Tyrosine	5.8 mg/g
Valine	3.0 mg/g

Components

Protein	22.5%
Carbohydrates	35.8%
Fat	30%
Moisture	5.7%
Ash	5.9%
Calories	503 per 100 g
Dietary fiber	35.1%
(3.0% soluble)	
Nitrogen-free extract	40.59

Polysaccharides

Carotene	7.63
International Units/gram	

Other Active Naturally Occurring Ingredients

(Hempseed Oil average % Main Fatty Acids) (76.78% of the Total Fat-Oil)

Linoleic (omega-6)	54.0
G-Linolenic (omega-6)	1.68
Linolenic (omega-3)	21.1

More on Hempseed Oil

Vitamin A	19,140 IU/kg
Insoluble Matter	0.01%
Chlorophyll	6 ppm
Free Fatty Acids	0.94%
Fat Stability AOM	5 hours
Phosphatides	0.03%
Unsaponified matter	0.28%
Saponification value	192.8
Melting point	(–8°C)
Flash Point	141°C
Smoke Point	165°C
Peroxide value	7.0 meg/kg
Moisture	19%
Specific Gravity	0.9295 @ 20°C

Fatty Acids in Hempseed Oil

	India	Cyprus	G.B.	Russia	Turkey	China
Percent Oil	30	36	31.4	34.1	35-38	42.4
Palmitic	7.4	9.5	9.5	6.5	9.4	7.3
Stearic	4.3	5.6	2	2.2	3.1	2.8
Oleic	13.1	10.8	7.8	12.9	14.9	11
Linoleic	54.4	54.4	56.2	57.1	49.2	53.2
Gamma-linolenic	n.s.	n.s.	n.s.	1.68*	n.s.	n.s.
Linolenic	19.5	18.7	22.4	19.7	23.1	23.2
Arachidic	1.2	1	1.9	n.s.	n.s.	1

*average of seven analyses, one showing 3% for this EFA.
n.s.= not stated

Sources

Jones, K. *Nutritional and Medicinal Guide to Hemp Seed.* Canada: Rainforest Botanical Laboratory, 1995.

Coconut

Coconut meat, raw

Nutritional value per 100 g (3.5 oz)

Energy	350 kcal
	1480 kJ
Carbohydrates	15.23 g
Sugars	6.23 g
Dietary fiber	9.0 g
Fat	33.49 g
Saturated	29.70 g
Monounsaturated	1.43 g
Polyunsaturated	0.37 g
Protein	3.3 g
Thiamin (Vit. B1)	0.066 mg 5%
Riboflavin (Vit. B2)	0.02 mg 1%
Niacin (Vit. B3)	0.54 mg 4%
Pantothenic acid (B5)	0.300 mg 6%
Vitamin B6	0.054 mg 4%
Folate (Vit. B9)	26 mg 7%
Vitamin C	3.3 mg 6%
Calcium	14 mg 1%
Iron	2.43 mg 19%
Magnesium	32 mg 9%
Phosphorus	113 mg 16%
Potassium	356 mg 8%
Zinc	1.1 mg 11%

(Percentages are relative to U.S. recommendations for adults.)

Source: USDA Nutrient Database for Standard

Amino Acid Content of Coconut Water

Amino Acid	mg/100g	mg/cup
Tryptophan	8	19
Threonine	26	62
Isoleucine	28	27
Leucine	53	127
Lysine	32	77
Methionine	13	31
Cystine	14	34
Phenylalanine	37	89
Tyrosine	22	53
Valine	44	106
Arginine	118	283
Histidine	17	41
Alanine	37	89
Aspartic Acid	70	168
Glutamic Acid	165	396
Glycine	34	82
Proline	30	72
Serine	37	89

Source: USDA National Nutrient Database for Standard

Note: Coconut water contains 18 amino acids. Sports drinks contain none.

Sugar Content in Juices

Juice (1 cup)	Sugar (g)	Calories (kcal)
Coconut Water	6.26	46
Vegetable Cocktail	7.99	46
Tomato	8.65	41
Carrot	9.23	94
Grapefruit	22.48	96
Orange	20.83	112
Apple	27.03	117
Pineapple	31.43	130
Grape	35.27	142

Source: USDA National Nutrient Database for Standard

Appendix I

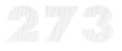

Nutrient Content in Gatorade, Powerade, and Coconut Water
(Value per 100 grams)

Nutrient	Units	Gatorade	Powerade	Coconut Water*
Sugar	g	5.33	6.02	3.71
Dietary Fiber	g	0	0	1.1
Calcium	mg	1	2	24
Iron	mg	0.20	0.25	0.29
Magnesium	mg	1	5	25
Phosphorus	mg	9	2	20
Potassium	mg	14	13	250
Sodium	mg	39	22	105
Zinc	mg	0.26	0.06	0.10
Copper	mg	0.25	0.25	0.04
Manganese	mg	0.05	0.05	0.142
Selenium	mcg	0.0	0.0	1
Fluoride	mcg	34	62	trace
Vitamin C	mg	0.4	0.4	2.4
Thiamin	mg	0.011	0.011	0.030
Niacin	mg	0.22	1.54	0.08
Pantothenic acid	mg	0.055	0.055	0.043
Vitamin B-6	mg	0.022	0.153	0.032
Folate	mcg	0.0	0.0	3
Amino Acids	mg	0.0	0.0	785

Unlike commercially produced beverages, natural products like coconut water do not have a precise chemical profile. All values listed here are averages of samples tested. These values will vary somewhat due to age, variety, and growing conditions.

Source: USDA National Nutrient Database for Standard

Fatty Acid Composition of Various Fats and Oils

Fatty Acid	Coco-nut	Palm Kernel	Palm	Butter	Lard	Beef	Soy-bean	Corn
Short-Chain Fatty Acid								
Butyric (C4:0)*	-	-	-	3	-	-	-	-
Caproic (C6:0)	0.5	-	-	1	-	-	-	-
Medium-Chain Fatty Acid								
Caprylic (C8:0)	7.8	4	-	1	-	-	-	-
Capric (C10:0)	6.7	4	-	3	-	-	-	-
Lauric (C12:0)	47.5	45	0.2	4	-	-	-	-
Long-Chain Fatty Acid								
Myristic (C14:0)	18.1	18	1.1	12	3	3.0	-	-
Palmitic (16:0)	8.8	9	44	29	24	29.0	11	11.5
Stearic (18:0)	2.6	3	4.5	11	18	22.0	4	2.2
Arachidic (C20:0)	0.1	-	-	5	1	-	-	-
Palmitoleic (C16:1)	-	-	0.1	4	-	-	-	-
Oleic (C18:1)	6.2	15	39.2	25	42	43.0	25	26.6
Linoleic (C18:2)	1.6	2	10.1	2	9	1.4	51	58.7
Linolenic (C18:3)	-	-	0.4		-	-	9	0.8
% saturated	92.1	83	45.2	69	46	54.0	15	13.7
% monounsaturated	6.2	15	39.3	29	42	43.0	25	26.6
%polyunsaturated	1.6	2	10.5	2	9	1.4	60	59.5

* The C indicates carbon atoms. The number after the C and before the colon indicates the number of carbon atoms in the fatty acid chain and the number after the colon the number of double bonds. A 0 after the colon is a saturated fat, a 1 after the colon is a monounsaturated fat, and a 2 or 3 indicates a polyunsaturated fat.

Source: Applewhite, T. H. (ed.) *Proceedings of the World Conference on Lauric Oils: Sources, Processing, and Applications.* Champaign, Illinois: ACOS Press, 1994.

Coconut Oil Antimicrobial Properties

Published medical studies show that MCFA's in coconut oil kill bacteria, fungi, and other organisms that cause the following illnesses and conditions:

Bacterial Infections

Throat and sinus infections
Urinary tract infections
Pneumonia
Ear infections
Rheumatic fever
Dental cavities and gum disease
Food poisoning
Toxic Shock Syndrome

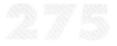
Meningitis
Gonorrhea
Pelvic inflammatory disease
Lymphogranuloma venereum
Conjunctivitis
Parrot fever
Gastric ulcers
Septicemia
Endocarditis
Enterocolitis

Viral Infections

Influenza
Measles
Herpes
Mononucleosis
Chronic Fatigue Syndrome
Hepatitis C
AIDS
SARS

Fungal Infections

Ringworm
Athlete's Foot
Jock Itch
Candidiasis
Diaper Rash
Thrush
Toenail Fungus

Parasite Infections

Giardiasis

Microorganisms Killed by Medium-Chain Fatty Acids (MCFAs)

Medical research has identified a number of pathogenic organisms that are inactivated by medium-chain fatty acids in coconut oil. Below is a listing of some of the organisms reported in the medical literature.

Viruses

Human Immunodeficiency Virus (HIV)
SARS coronavirus
Measles virus
Rubeola virus
Herpes simplex virus (HSV-1 and -2)
Herpes viridae
Sarcoma virus
Syncytial virus
Human lymphotropic virus (Type 1)
Vesicular stomatitis virus (VSV)
Visna virus
Cytomegalovirus (CMV)
Epstein-Barr virus
Influenza virus
Leukema virus
Pneumonovirus
Hepatitis C virus
Coxsackie B4 virus

Bacteria

Listeria monocytogenes
Helicobacter pylori
Hemophilis influenza
Staphylococcus aureus
Staphylococcus epidermidis
Streptococcus agalactiae
Escherichia coli
Pseudomonas aeruginosa
Acinetobacter aeruginosa
Acinetobacter baumannii
Neisseria
Chlamydia tracchomatis
Steptococci Groups A, B, F, & G
Gram-positive organisms
Gram-negative organisms
(if pretreated with chelator)

Parasites

Giardia
Ciliate protozoa

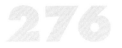

Toxins Mitigated by Coconut Oil

Studies show that coconut oil tempers or blocks the harmful effects of many toxins including the following:

Ethanol
MSG
N-nitrosomethylurea
Azoxymethane
Benzpyrene
Azaserine
Diamethylbenzanthracene
Dimethylhydrazine
Dimethynitrosamine
Methylmethanesulfonate
Tetracycline
Streptococci endotoxin/exotoxin
Staphylococci endotoxin/exotoxin
E. coli endotoxin
Aflatoxin

Sources

Fife, B. *Coconut Cures*. Colorado Springs, CO: Piccadilly Books, 2005.

———. *Coconut Water*. Colorado Springs, CO: Piccadilly Books, 2008.

Appendix II
Scientific Studies

Goji Berry
Scientific Journal References

INCREASES ENERGY

International Journal of Biological Macromolecules, June 2008, Vol.42 Issue 5, p. 447–449

"Protective effect of Lycium barbarum polysaccharides on oxidative damage in skeletal muscles of exhaustive exercise rats. In conclusion, L. barbarum polysaccharides administration can significantly decrease the oxidative stress induced by the exhaustive exercise."

ROOT BARK VS. DIABETES

Therapy, Sept. 2007, Vol. 4 Issue 5, p. 547–553

"Effects of Lycium barbarum L. root bark extract on alloxan-induced diabetic mice. The results indicate that LbL administration to diabetic mice would alleviate the increases in blood glucose and lipid levels associated with diabetes, improve abnormal glucose metabolism and increase insulin secretion by restoring the impaired pancreas β-cells in alloxan-induced diabetic mice. This would suggest that LbL has hypoglycemic and hypolipidemic potential and could be useful for diabetic therapy."

NEUROLOGICAL PROTECTION

Brain Research, July 2007, Vol. 1158, p. 123–134

"Characterizing the neuroprotective effects of alkaline extract of Lycium barbarum on β-amyloid peptide neurotoxicity. Taken together, our results suggested that the glycoconjugate isolated from novel alkaline extraction method can open up a new avenue for drug discovery in neurodegenerative diseases."

Experimental Gerontology, Aug. 2005, Vol. 40 Issue 8/9, p. 716–727

"Neuroprotective effects of anti-aging oriental medicine Lycium barbarum against β-amyloid peptide neurotoxicity. Taken together, we have proved our hypothesis by showing neuroprotective effects of the extract from L. barbarum. Study on anti-aging herbal medicine like L. barbarum may open a new therapeutic window for the prevention of neurodegenerative diseases."

LONGEVITY
Journal of Ethnopharmacology, May 2007, Vol. 111 Issue 3, p. 504–511

"Effect of the Lycium barbarum polysaccharides on age-related oxidative stress in aged mice. It is concluded that the Lycium barbarum polysaccharides can be used in compensating the decline in TAOC, immune function and the activities of antioxidant enzymes and thereby reduces the risks of lipid peroxidation accelerated by age-induced free radical."

ANTIOXIDANTS
Carbohydrate Polymers, May 2007, Vol. 69 Issue 1, p. 172–178

"Inhibition of Lycium barbarum polysaccharides and Ganoderma lucidum polysaccharides against oxidative injury by y-irradiation in rat liver mitochondria. The inhibitory effects of GLP, at the entire concentration range, are stronger than LBP. Moreover, the two polysaccharides are more effective that α-tocopherol (VE) in inhibiting irradiation-induced oxidative injury. Hence, our results indicate that GLP and LBP have potent antioxidant properties in vitro in mitochondrial membranes of rat liver."

International Journal of Biological Macromolecules, April 2007, Vol. 40 Issue 5, p. 461–465

"Protective effect of Lycium barbarum polysaccharides on streptozotocin-induced oxidative stress in rats. Therefore, we may assume that LBP is effective in the protection of liver and kidney tissue from the damage of STZ-induced diabetic rats and that the LBP may be of use as a antihyperglycemia agent."

Journal of Ethnopharmacology, Oct. 2002, Vol. 82 Issue 2/3, p. 169

"Protective effect of Frustuc Lycii polysaccharides against time and hyperthermia-induced damage in cultured seminiferous epithelium. Together, these results demonstrate the protective effect of FLPS on time- and hyperthermia-induced testicular degeneration in vitro, indicate the potential mechanism of action for this protective effect, and provide effect, and provide a scientific basis for the traditional use of this plant."

IMPROVES EYESIGHT
Experimental Neurology, Jan. 2007, Vol. 203 Issue 1, p. 269–273

"Neuroprotective effects of Lycium barbarum Lynn on protecting retinal ganglion cells in an ocular hypertension model of glaucoma. In conclusion, this is the first in vivo report showing the therapeutic function of L. barbarum against neurodegeneration in the retina of rat OH model. The results demonstrate that this extract may be a potential candidate for the development of neuroprotective drug against the loss of RGCs in glaucoma."

INCREASES FERTILITY AND SEXUAL FUNCTION
Life Sciences, July 2006, Vol. 79 Issue 7, p. 613–621

"Lycium barbarum polysaccharides: Protective effects against heat-induced

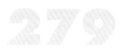
damage of rat testes and HO induced DNA damage in mouse testicular cells and beneficial effect on sexual behavior and reproductive function. LBP improved the copulatory performance and reproductive function of hemicastrated male rats, such as shortened penis erection latency and mount latency, regulated secretion of sexual hormones and increased hormone levels, raised accessory sexual organ weights, and improved sperm quantity and quality. The present findings support the folk reputation of L. barbarum fruits as an aphrodisiac and fertility-facilitating agent, and provide scientific evidence for a basis for the extensive use of L. barbarum fruits as a traditional remedy for male infertility in China."

IMPROVES CARDIOVASCULAR HEALTH (CACAO AND GOJI)

Agricultural Research, Jan. 2006, Vol. 54 Issue 1, p. 22

"Plant Compounds Inhibit Blood Clotting. Synthesized were the natural compounds N-caffeoyldopamine and N-coumaroyldopamine and their analogs, which are found in sweet peppers, Chinese wolfberry (goji berry), and cocoa. Based on Park's findings, the compounds significantly suppress an adhesive molecule, P-selectin, that glues platelets to white blood cells and blood vessel walls."

IMPROVES IMMUNE SYSTEM

Cancer Biotherapy and Radiopharmaceuticals, April 2005, Vol. 20 Issue 2, p. 155–162

"Therapeutic Effects of Lycium barbarum Polysaccharide (LBP) on Irradiation or Chemotherapy-Induced Myelosuppresive mice. All dosages of LBP significantly enhanced peripheral PLT counts of chemotherapy-induced myelosuppresive mice on days 7."

Journal of Experimental Therapeutics & Oncology, 2004, Vol. 4 Issue 3, p. 181–187

"Therapeutic effects of Lycium barbarum polysaccharide (LBP) on mitomycin C (MMC)-induced myelosuppresive mice. LBP showed no obviously effect on neutropenia induced in mice by MMC. Conclusion: LBP is effective on peripheral RBC and PLT recovery of MMC-induced myelosuppresive mice."

PROTECTS LIVER

Life Sciences, March 2005, Vol. 76 Issue 18, p. 2115–2124

"Effect of lycium barbarum polysaccharide on human hepatoma cells: Inhibition of proliferation and induction of apoptosis. Moreover, the distribution of calcium in cells was changed. Taken together, the study suggests that the induction of cell cycle arrest and the increase of intracellular calcium in apoptotic system may participate in the antiproliferative activity of LBP in QGY7703 cells."

Journal of Ethnopharmacology, Jan. 2005, Vol. 96 Issue 3, p. 529–535

"Protective effect of Lycium chinense fruit on carbon tetrachloride-induced hepatotoxicity. Based on these results, it was suggested that the hepatoprotective effects of the LFE might be related to antioxidative activity and expressional regulation of CYP2E1."

Bioorganic & Medicinal Chemistry Letters, Jan. 2003, Vol. 13 Issue 1, p. 79

"Hepatoprotective pyrrole derivatives of Lycium chinense fruits. These compounds and a related synthetic methylated compound (4) were evaluated for their biological activity and structure–activity relationship, and compounds 1 and 2 showed hepatoprotective effects comparable to silybin at the concentration of 0.1 μM."

PROTECTS AGAINST CANCER

European Journal of Pharmacology, June 2003, Vol. 471 Issue 3, p. 217

"A polysaccharide-protein complex from Lycium barbarum upregulates cytokine expression in human peripheral blood mononuclear cells. Administration of LBP 3p increased the expression of interleukin-2 and tumor necrosis factor-α at both mRNA and protein levels in a dose-dependent manner. The results suggest that LBP 3p may induce immune responses and possess potential therapeutic efficacy in cancer."

GROW MEDICINAL MUSHROOMS ON GOJI BERRY EXTRACT

Food Chemistry, Sept. 2008, Vol. 110 Issue 2, p. 446–4453

"Effect of Lycium barbarum extract on production and immunomodulatory activity of the extracellular polysaccharopeptides from submerged fermentation culture of Coriolus versicolor. Moreover, the ePSP from C. versicolor cultured with supplementary L. barbarum extract exhibits significant immunomodulatory activity as judged by its effects on the production of nitric oxide and several cytokines by murine RAW264.7 macrophages."

GOJI LEAF IS A PREBIOTIC

Bioresource Technology, March 2008, Vol. 99 Issue 5, p. 1383–1393

"Effects of Chinese wolfberry (Lycium chinense P. Mill.) leaf hydrolysates on the growth of Pediococcus acidilactici. The growth-enhancing effects of LYCH leaf hydrolysates indicate the potential of developing new applications for LYCH leaves in promoting the growth of other probiotic cells using a simple process."

ESSENTIAL SUGARS

European Polymer Journal, Feb. 2007, Vol. 43 Issue 2, p. 488–497

"Evaluation of antioxidant activity of the polysaccharides extracted from Lycium barbarum fruits in vitro. Analysis shows that its carbohydrate content is up to 97.54% mainly composed of:

d-rhamnose	d-xylose
d-arabinose	d-fucose
d-glucose	d-galactose

The data obtained in the in vitro models clearly establish the antioxidant potency of the polysaccharides extracted from L. barbarum fruits."

FAT COMPOSITION

Chemistry of Natural Compounds, Jan. 2006, Vol. 42 Issue 1, p. 24–25
"Composition of the essential oils of Lycium barbarum and L. ruthenicum fruits. The main component in the oil of L. barbarum were found to be hexadecanoic acid, linoleic acid, β-elemene, myristic acid, and ethyl hexadecanoate. The essential oil of L. ruthenicum has heptocosane, ethyl linoleate, hexacosane, nonacosane, and ethyl hexadecanoate as the main compounds."

FLAVONOIDS

Food Chemistry, Sept. 2004, Vol. 87 Issue 2, p. 283
"The efficiency of flavonoids in polar extracts of Lycium chinense Mill fruits as free radical scavenger. The main flavonoids in Lycium chinense Mill fruits were rutin and chlorogenic acid in water extract, rutin and protocatechuic acid 50% ethanol extract and rutin in 95% ethanol extract as determined with high-performance liquid chromatography. The antiradical efficiency of the extracts tended to become stronger as the polarity of the solvents decreased."

Additional Goji Berry References
BOOKS

Benson, L., and R. Darrow. March *Trees and Shrubs of the Southwestern Deserts.* University of Arizona and University of New Mexico, 1954.

Gross, P. M., X. Zhang, and R. Zhang. *Wolfberry: Nature's Bounty of Nutrition and Health.* Charleston, SC: Booksurge Publishing, 2006.

Mindell, Earl, and Rick Handel. *Goji: the Himalayan Health Secret.* Texas: Momentum Media, 2003.

Teeguarden, R. *The Ancient Wisdom of the Chinese Tonic Herbs.* New York: Warner Books, Inc., 1998.

Vines, Robert A. *Trees, Shrubs, and Woody Wines of the Southwest.* Austin, TX: University of Texas Press, 1960.

Cacao

CHOCOLATE BETTER THAN KISSING

When it comes to tongues, melting chocolate is better than a passionate kiss, scientists have found. Couples in their twenties had their heart rates and brains monitored while they first melted chocolate in their mouths and then kissed.

Chocolate caused a more intense and longer lasting "buzz" than kissing, and doubled volunteers' heart rates.

The researchers compared their resting heart rates with those during the chocolate and kissing tests.

Although kissing set the heart pounding, the effect did not last as long as that seen with the chocolate, which increased heart rates from a resting rate of about 60 beats per minute to 140.

Source: http://news.bbc.co.uk/2/hi/health/6558775.stm

CHOCOLATE AND SEX

Dr. Andrea Salonia, an Italian researcher, says he has found an association between eating chocolate and sexual fulfillment. Women who love chocolate, he says, seem to have better love lives.

Salonia's group at the San Raffaele Hospital in Milan had 153 women fill out standard female sexual function questionnaires, among other lifestyle and psychological indices. The women were between 26 and 44 years old, with a median age of 35. It turned out that 120 women, average age 35, reported they ate chocolate frequently, compared with 33 women whose average age was 40.4.

Both overall sexual function and sexual desire were significantly greater among the chocolate-eaters than among those in the older group who were more likely to spurn chocolate, said Salonia.

Source: Bloom, Mark. Healthday, www.healthday.com. Dec. 5–8, 2004, London: presentation, European Society for Sexual Medicine annual meeting.

CHOCOLATE IS GOOD FOR THE HEART

Norman Hollenberg from Harvard Medical School and Brigham and Women's Hospital presented new data, also published in the current issue of the *International Journal of Medical Sciences,* where he used death certificates to compare the cause of death of island-dwelling Kuna to those who live on mainland Panama, who do not regularly drink the flavonol-rich cocoa.

Hollenberg reported that the relative risk of death from heart disease on the Panama mainland was 1,280 percent higher than on the islands and death from cancer was 630 percent higher, compared to the islanders.

Source: Bayard, V., F. Chamorro, J. Motta, N. K. Hollenberg. "Does flavonol intake influence mortality from nitric oxide-dependent processes? Ischemic heart disease, stroke, diabetes mellitus, and cancer in Panama." *International Journal of Medical Sciences.* Volume 4 (2007), pp. 53–58.

CHOCOHOLICS REJOICE! MORE BENEFITS FOUND IN HEART STUDY

Chocolate lovers who flunked out of a Johns Hopkins University study on aspirin and heart disease helped researchers stumble on an explanation of why a little chocolate a day can cut the risk of heart attack.

It turns out chocolate, like aspirin, affects the platelets that cause blood to clot, Diane Becker of the Johns Hopkins University's School of Medicine and her colleagues discovered.

"What these chocolate offenders taught us is that the chemical in cocoa beans has a biochemical effect similar to aspirin in reducing platelet clumping, which can be fatal if a clot forms and blocks a blood vessel, causing a heart attack," Becker said in a telephone interview.

Source: Reuters, November 14, 2006.

CHOCOLATE ANTIOXIDANTS

The health benefits of epicatechin, a compound found in cocoa, are so striking that it may rival penicillin and anesthesia in terms of importance to public health, reports Marina Murphy in *Chemistry & Industry,* the magazine of the SCI. Norman Hollenberg, professor of medicine at Harvard Medical School, told *C&I* that epicatechin is so important that it should be considered a vitamin.

Hollenberg has spent years studying the benefits of cocoa drinking on the Kuna people in Panama. He found that the risk of 4 of the 5 most common killer diseases: stroke, heart failure, cancer, and diabetes, is reduced to less then 10 percent in the Kuna. They can drink up to 40 cups of cocoa a week. Natural cocoa has high levels of epicatechin.

Note: This story has been adapted from a news release issued by *Society of Chemical Industry.*

Source: "Cocoa 'Vitamin' Health Benefits Could Outshine Penicillin." *Science Daily.*

CHOCOLATE LOWERS BLOOD PRESSURE

A chocolate treat may be better than green or black tea at keeping high blood pressure in check.

A new study suggests that dark chocolate and other cocoa-rich products may be better at lowering blood pressure than tea.

Researchers compared the blood pressure-lowering effects of cocoa and tea in previously published studies and found eating cocoa-rich foods was associated with an average 4.7-point lower systolic blood pressure (the top number in a blood pressure reading) and 2.8-point lower diastolic blood pressure (the bottom number). But no such effect was found among any of the studies on black or green tea.

Cocoa and tea are both rich in a class of antioxidants known as polyphenols. But researchers say they contain different types of polyphenols, and those in cocoa may be more effective at lowering blood pressure.

Source: Warner, Jennifer. "Dark Chocolate, Other Cocoa-Rich Foods May Lower Blood Pressure Better Than Tea." *WebMD Medical News* (April 9, 2007). Reviewed by Louise Chang, MD.

POLYPHENOLS HELP BLOOD PRESSURE

In their review, researchers reviewed the effects of cocoa-rich products, such as dark chocolate or specially formulated polyphenol-rich milk chocolate, and blood pressure in five studies, which totaled 173 participants and lasted on average two weeks. They also reviewed black and green tea and blood pressure in five different studies that totaled 343 participants and lasted on average four weeks. All studies were published between 1966 and 2006.

"We believe that any dietary advice must account for the high sugar, fat, and calorie intake with most cocoa products," write researcher Dirk Taubert, MD, PhD, of the University Hospital of Cologne in Germany, and colleagues, in the Archives of Internal Medicine. "Rationally applied, cocoa products might be considered part of dietary approaches to lower hypertension risk."

Source: Taubert, D.. News Release. *Archives of Internal Medicine* 167 (2007): 626–34.

DARK CHOCOLATE IS BETTER FOR LOWERING BLOOD PRESSURE

Dark chocolate—but not white chocolate—may help reduce blood pressure and boosts the body's ability to metabolize sugar from food, according to the results of a small study.

Investigators from the University of L'Aquila in Italy found that after eating only 100 grams, or 3.5 ounces, of dark chocolate every day for 15 days, 15 healthy people had lower blood pressures and were more sensitive to insulin, an important factor in metabolizing sugar.

In contrast, eating roughly the same amount of white chocolate for the same period of time did not affect either blood pressure or insulin sensitivity.

Other research validates that when it comes to chocolate, type does matter. One study found that eating milk chocolate did little to raise antioxidant levels in the blood, perhaps because milk interferes with the absorption of antioxidants from chocolate.

Another study showed that elderly people with high blood pressure experienced a drop in pressure after eating dark chocolate bars, but not white chocolate, which contains no flavonoids.

Source: McCook, Alison. "When It Comes to Chocolate, Order Dark, Not White." *American Journal of Clinical Nutrition,* as reported by Reuters Health (March 21, 2005).

CHOCOLATE IMPROVES MENTAL PERFORMANCE

A new study hints that eating milk chocolate may boost brain function. "Chocolate contains many substances that act as stimulants, such as theobromine, phenethylamine, and caffeine," Dr. Bryan Raudenbush from Wheeling Jesuit University in West Virginia noted in comments to Reuters Health.

"These substances by themselves have previously been found to increase alertness and attention and what we have found is that by consuming chocolate you can get the stimulating effects, which then lead to increased mental performance."

To study the effects of various chocolate types on brain power, Raudenbush and colleagues had a group of volunteers consume, on four separate occasions, 85 grams of milk chocolate; 85 grams of dark chocolate; 85 grams of carob; and nothing (the control condition).

After a 15-minute digestive period, participants completed a variety of computer-based neuropsychological tests designed to assess cognitive performance including memory, attention span, reaction time, and problem solving.

"Composite scores for verbal and visual memory were significantly higher for milk chocolate than the other conditions," Raudenbush told Reuters. And consumption of milk and dark chocolate was associated with improved impulse control and reaction time.

Previous research has shown that some nutrients in food aid in glucose release and increased blood flow, which may augment cognitive performance. The current findings, said Raudenbush, "provide support for nutrient release via chocolate consumption to enhance cognitive performance."

Source: Reuters, May 25, 2006.

CACAO VERSUS DIABETES

Dietary supplementation with cacao liquor proanthocyanidins (CLPr) reduced blood glucose levels in obese diabetic mice, and may offer human diabetics significant benefits, says a new study from Japan.

"Dietary supplementation with CLPr can dose-dependently prevent the development of hyperglycaemia in diabetic obese mice," wrote lead author Makoto Tomaru in the journal Nutrition. "The dietary intake of food or drinks produced from cacao beans might be beneficial in preventing the onset of type-2 diabetes mellitus."

The potential health benefits of cocoa have been gaining increasing interest, with studies reporting that flavonoid-rich chocolate may reduce the risk of cardiovascular disease. However, according to Tomaru and co-workers, this is the first study to report that CLPr can prevent aggravation of type-2 diabetes mellitus.

Source: M. Tomura, H. Takano, N. Osakabe, A. Yasuda, K. I. Inoue, R. Yanagisawa, T. Ohwatari, and H. Uematsu. "Dietary supplementation with cacao liquor proanthocyanidins prevents elevation of blood glucose levels in diabetic obese mice." *Nutrition* (Elsevier) Published online ahead of print, doi: 10.1016/j.nut.2007.01.007

CACAO INCREASES LONGEVITY

At five-year intervals over a 15-year period, 470 men aged over 65 were questioned about their dietary intake of cocoa and received physical examinations. The men were placed in three groups according to their level of cocoa consumption and data about their health was collected. During the study, 314 men died, 152 due to cardiovascular disease.

"The men in the group that consumed the least cocoa were twice as likely to die from a heart attack than those in the group that consumed the most cocoa—at least 4g per day—and the risk remained lower even when other factors such as smoking, physical exercise, and weight were taken into account," said lead researcher Brian Buijsse, at the Dutch National Institute for Public Health and the Environment.

He added: "And men in the study who consumed the most cocoa were less likely to die of any cause."

The high-cocoa men also had significantly lower blood pressure than the other groups—but Buijsse said that the link between low blood pressure and reduced risk of cardiovascular disease cannot be made from his results. Instead, he says that cocoa-containing antioxidant chemicals, called flavonols, may be the cause.

Source: "Eating Chocolate May Halve Risk of Dying." *Archives of Internal Medicine* 166: 411, as cited by NewScientist.com news service 21:00 27 February 2006, Gaia Vince http://www.newscientist.com/channel/health/dn8780.html

CHOCOLATE PROTECTS THE SKIN

German researchers have shown that ingesting cocoa solids and flavonoids—dark chocolate—can fight skin cancer. Their findings are preliminary because they come from a trial of just 24 women who were recruited to add cocoa to their breakfasts every day for about 3 months.

Half the women drank hot cocoa containing a hefty dose of flavonoids, natural plant-based antioxidants that research has suggested prevent heart attacks. The remaining volunteers got cocoa that looked and tasted the same but that had relatively little of the flavonoids. At the beginning and end of the trial, Wilhelm Stahl of Heinrich-Heine University in Düsseldorf and his colleagues conducted a host of tests on each volunteer. One assessment involved irradiating each woman's skin with slightly more ultraviolet (UV) light than had turned her skin red before the trial began.

The skin of the women who had received the flavonoid-rich cocoa did not redden nearly as much as did the skin of recruits who had drunk the flavonoid-poor beverage. Women getting the abundant flavonoids also had skin that was smoother and moister than that of the other women.

Source: Raloff, Janet. "Chocolate as Sunscreen."
    http://www.sciencenews.org/articles/20060617/food.asp.

CHOCOLATE DOES NOT CAUSE ACNE

Two seminal studies continue to prove that chocolate does not cause acne. The National Institutes of Health now states that "despite the popular belief that chocolate, nuts, and other foods cause acne, this does not seem to be true."

In one of the studies, at the University of Pennsylvania, a group of acne patients was given a bar of "chocolate" liquor (the substance that's the base for all chocolate products) resembling a chocolate bar and had 28 percent vegetable fat to imitate the fat content of chocolate liquor and cocoa butter. Another group got real chocolate in a test bar with almost ten times as much chocolate liquor as a normal 1.4-ounce bar.

The acne neither improved nor worsened with the chocolate or the placebo.

In the other study, 80 midshipmen with acne at the U.S. Naval Academy were divided into chocolate abstainers and chocolate-eaters. After a month, careful observation showed no changes in their acne.

Source: Engler, Mary, Jeffrey Blumberg, and Jean Mayer. *Journal of the American College of Nutrition* (June 2004).

CHOCOLATE IS GOOD FOR OUR TEETH

A bar of chocolate a day might keep the dentist away, according to new research into the cavity-fighting properties of cocoa. Researchers at Tulane University in New Orleans, Louisiana, have discovered that cocoa powder contains an extract that is more effective than fluoride in fighting cavities and protecting dental health.

The compound is a white, crystalline powder commonly found in chocolate. It's chemical composition is similar to that of caffeine and, in tests carried out at the university, it was found to harden tooth enamel.

The team, led by doctoral student Arman Sadeghpour, compared the cocoa-based substance with fluoride in tests carried out on the enamel of human teeth. The results were used to create a toothpaste which incorporates the cocoa.

Source: Boal, Catherine. "Cocoa Extract more Effective than Fluoride."

CACAO SKIN FIGHTS CAVITIES

By using an extract of husk of cacao, obtained with a polar solvent, Lotte Co. Ltd. of Tokyo, Japan, believes it has come up with a composition for inhibiting sordes formation and thereby cutting down on tooth decay.

The buildup of sordes on the teeth, and the subsequent destruction of the tooth enamel by microorganisms contained in the sordes, is believed to be caused by the conversion of sucrose in food to the viscous polysaccharide, glucan, as a result of the activity of glucosyltransferase, which is an extracellular enzyme of streptococcus mutans. Glucan is the substance that causes sordes buildup.

Source: Biomedical Materials. February 1, 1990.
   http://static.highbeam.com/b/biomedicalmaterials/february011990/cacaoextract-couldcutdownontoothdecay/

Additional Cacao References

BOOKS

Coe, Sophie D., Coe, Michael D. *The True History of Chocolate.* New York: Thames and Hudson, 1996.

Dahl, Roald. *Charlie and the Chocolate Factory.* New York: Puffin Books, 1964.

Foster, Nelson, Cordell, Linda S. *Chilies to Chocolate: Food the Americas Gave the World.* Tucson, AZ: University of Arizona Press, 1992.

Kilham, Chris. *Psyche Delicacies: Coffee, Chocolate, Chiles, Kava, and Cannabis, and Why They're Good For You.* Emmaus, PA: Rodale Press, 2001

Lopez, Ruth. *Chocolate: The Nature of Indulgence.* New York: Harry N. Abrams, 2002.

McFadden, Christine, France, Christine. *Chocolate: Cooking with the World's Best Ingredient.* London: Hermes House, 1997.

Pendell, Dale. *Pharmakodynamis: Stimulating Plants, Potions & Herbcraft.* San Francisco: Mercury House, 2002.

Presilla, Maricel E. *The New Taste of Chocolate: A Cultural and Natural History of Cacao with Recipes.* Berkeley, CA: Ten Speed Press, 2001.

Wolfe, David, and Shazzie. *Naked Chocolate.* Berkeley: North Atlantic Books, 2005.

Young, Allen M. *The Chocolate Tree: A Natural History of Cacao.* Washington, D.C.: Smithsonian Institution Press, 1994.

WEB SITES

http://www.sacredchocolate.com

Maca

Scientific Journal References

HUMAN STUDY SHOWS LIBIDO AND SPERM INCREASE

The first known published human study on maca's effect on fertility and libido in men was conducted through the department of Physiological Sciences, University Peruana Cayetano Heredia, in Lima, Peru. The study, published in the *Asian Journal of Andrology,* involved 9 healthy men (aged 22–24) who completed the 4-month trial with gelatinized maca. Either 1,500 or 3,000 mg. was administered orally each day. Study data showed that maca: (Gonzales)

- Increased sexual desire (libido) by 180%
- Increased number and mobility of sperm
- Increased DHEA levels in a majority of the men
- Decreased anxiety and stress
- Increased adrenal androgen (adrenaline)
- Promotes glucose utilization for energy rather than being processed into fat storage
- Produced a "general sense of well-being"
- Lowered blood pressure (diastolic)
- Balanced blood iron levels

Experiments with men as well as with animals show not only greater seminal volume by 20 percent, but also sperm quality, more than 184 percent increased spermatozoon, and more than 208 percent improved mobility, leading to enhanced fertility. (Gonzales) Other studies also demonstrate broods increasing by 25 to 40 percent in dogs, cows, sheep, and other animals. (Chacón)

In female animals, maca consumption significantly increased Graaf follicles, and other favorable endometrium characteristics, which indicates a higher fertility level.

Source: Ley, B.M. *MACA: Adaptogen and Hormonal Regulator.*

LIBIDO

Maca also helps improve sexual activity and satisfaction by increasing vaginal lubrication in women as well as increasing seminal volume (ejaculate) by 30 percent in men.

In the prestigious medical journal *Urology* (April 2000), scientists tell of the experience of rats with erectile disorder were fed maca compared to controls. The maca group had 400 percent more copulation than the controls.

Maca provides a means of normalizing our steroid hormones like testosterone, progesterone, and estrogen. Therefore, it facilitates balance to the hormonal changes of aging. In men, it restores a healthy functional status in which they experience a more active libido.

Source: Ley, B.M. *MACA: Adaptogen and Hormonal Regulator.*

SAFETY AND SIDE EFFECTS OF MACA

Maca is considered to be a "warming herb" according to Chinese medicine, and therefore should be used with caution by those with high blood pressure. However, this has not been tested scientifically.

Toxicity studies conducted in at Product Safety Labs of East Brunswick, N.J., showed absolutely no toxicity, and no adverse pharmacological affects of maca.

Based on its long history of use as a medicinal supplement and as a food, maca

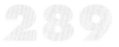
appears to be safe. The following are structure/function statements permitted under section 6 of DSHEA (Dietary Supplemental Health and Education Act) for maca:

- Increases energy, stamina, and mental clarity
- Supports the thyroid
- Supports normal sexual function
- Promotes hormone balance

Source: Ley, B. M. *MACA: Adaptogen and Hormonal Regulator.*

RED MACA

Red maca has the same nutritional profile and all of the same beneficial properties as regular (white, yellow, or black) maca, but it appears to possess additional properties of its own that may be more beneficial to mens' health.

As a result of recent scientific studies, red maca has been proposed to have important implications in the treatment of prostate diseases, including prostate cancer. Phytochemical analyses showed red maca to have greater amounts of the compounds responsible for antioxidant and antitumor activity than other types of maca.

Source: Gonzales, Gustavo F., Sara Miranda, Jessica Nieto, Gilma Fernández, Sandra Yucra, Julio Rubio, Pedro Yi, and Manuel Gasco. "Red maca (Lepidium meyenii) reduced prostate size." *Reproductive Biology and Endocrinology;* 3 (2005):5.

Additional Maca References

BOOKS

Chacón, G. "La Maca (Lepidium peruvianum) Chacón sp. Nov. Y su habitat." *Revista Peruana de Biologia* 3 (1990): 171–272.

———. "Estudio fitoquimico de Lepidium meyenii." Dissertation, Univ., Nac. Mayo de San Marcos, Peru.

———. *Maca (Lepidium peruvianum Chacón) Millenarian Peruvian Food with Highly Nutritional Properties.* Lima, Peru, 2001.

Gonzales, G. F. "A test for bioandrogenicity in men attending an infertility service." *Arch Androl.* 21 (1988): 135–42.

———. "Functional structure and ultra structure of seminal vesicles." *Arch Androl.* 22 (1988): 1–13.

Gonzales, G. F., A. Cordova, C. Gonzales, and A. Chung. "Lepidium meyenii (Maca) improved semen parameters in adult men." *Asian J Androl* 3 (1988): 301–3.

Gonzales, G.F., Ruiz A., Gonzales C., Villegas L., Cordova A. 2001. "Effect of Lepidium meyenii (Maca) roots on spermatogenesis of male rats." *Asian J Androl.* Sep; 3(3) p. 231–3.

Johns, Timothy. *The Origins of Human Diet and Medicine.* Tucson: University of Arizona Press, 1990.

Ley, B. M. *MACA: Adaptogen and Hormonal Regulator.* Minnesota: BL Publications, 2003.

Zheng, B.L., He, K., Kim, C.H., et al. "Effect of lipidic extract from Lepidium meyenii on sexual behavior in mice and rats." *Urology* 55 (2000): 598–602.

WEB SITES

http://en.wikipedia.org/wiki/Adaptogen

http://www.pfaf.org/database/plants.php?Lepidium+meyenii

Bee Products

Scientific Journal Reference

Honey, used in tea or hot water in Canada for generations to soothe sore throats, could soon be substituted for antibiotics in fighting stubborn ear, nose, and throat infections, according to a new study.

Ottawa University doctors found in tests that ordinary honey kills bacteria that cause sinus infections, and does it better in most cases than antibiotics.

"It's astonishing," researcher Joseph Marson said of bees' unexplained ability to combine the nectar of flowers into a seemingly potent medicine.

The preliminary tests were conducted in laboratory dishes, not in live patients, but included the "superbug" methicillin-resistant Staphylococcus aureus or MRSA, which is highly resistant to antibiotics.

Source: "Early Study Touts Honey As Antibiotics Substitute." Sept. 24, 2008.
  http://ca.news.yahoo.com/s/afp/080924/health/canada_medicine_research

Additional Bee Products References

BOOKS

Buxton, Simon. *The Shamanic Way Of The Bee.* Rochester, VT: Destiny, 2006.

Jensen, Bernard. *Bee Well, Bee Wise with Bee Pollen, Bee Propolis, Royal Jelly.* Escondido, CA: Bernard Jensen, 1993.

Kacera, Walter. *Pollen Power, Nectar of Life.* 2002.

Traynor, Joe. *Honey, The Gourmet Medicine.* Bakersfield, CA: Kovak Books, 2002.

ARTICLES

"Fresh Royal Jelly" by Y.S. Royal Jelly and Honey Farm (available on the web site: www.yahwehsaliveandwell.com)

"Bee Propolis: Nature's Healing Balm With Immune Boosting Properties" by Katherine East (available on the web site: www.naturalnews.com)

WEB SITES

http://homepages.ihug.com.au/~panopus/parachemy/parachemyvii2.htm

http://www2.wcoil.com/

http://www.durhamsbeefarm.com/beepollen.htm

http://www.shirleys-wellness-cafe.com/bee.htm

http://www.alternativescentral.com/phf2a-beepollen.htm

http://thehoneybees.com/pollen.html

Spirulina
Scientific Journal References

Adding spirulina to cultured immune system cells significantly increases the production of infection fighting cytokines, say immunologists at UC Davis School of Medicine and Medical Center. Their finding is published in the Fall issue of the *Journal of Medicinal Foods*.

"We found that nutrient-rich spirulina is a potent inducer of interferon-gamma (13.6-fold increase) and a moderate stimulator of both interleukin-4 and interleukin-1beta (3.3-fold increase)," says Eric Gershwin, professor and chief of the Division of Rheumatology, Allergy, and Clinical Immunology at UC Davis. "Together, increases in these cytokines suggest that spirulina is a strong proponent for protecting against intracellular pathogens and parasites and can potentially increase the expression of agents that stimulate inflammation, which also helps to protect the body against infectious and potentially harmful microorganisms."

To evaluate the effects of spirulina on the immune system, the UC Davis immunologists collected blood samples from 12 healthy volunteers, separating out the peripheral blood mononuclear cells. These cells, which include macrophages, monocytes, and lymphocytes, including B and T cells, work as a team to mount an immune response. The researchers incubated these cell cultures with dilutions of spirulina made from 429 mg capsules of dried, powdered spirulina.

Source: "UC Davis Study Shows Spirulina Boosts Immune System." December 1, 2000.
http://news.ucdmc.ucdavis.edu/spirulina_study.html.

In April 1996, scientists from the Laboratory of Viral Pathogenesis, Dana-Farber Cancer Institute, and Harvard Medical School and Earthrise Farms, Calipatria, California, announced ongoing research, saying, "Water extract of Spirulina platensis inhibits HIV-1 replication in human derived T-cell lines and in human peripheral blood mononuclear cells. A concentration of 5–10 mg/ml was found to reduce viral production." HIV-1 is the AIDS virus. Small amounts of spirulina extract reduced viral replication while higher concentrations totally stopped its reproduction. Importantly, with the therapeutic index of >100, spirulina extract was nontoxic to human cells at concentrations stopping viral replication.

Another group of medical scientists has published new studies regarding a purified water extract unique to spirulina named calcium-spirulan. It inhibits replication of HIV-1, herpes simplex, human cytomegalovirus, influenza A virus, mumps virus and measles virus in-vitro, yet is very safe for human cells. It protects human and monkey cells from viral infection in cell culture. According to peer-reviewed scientific journal reports this extract, "holds great promise for treatment of ... HIV-1, HSV-1, and HCM infections, which is particularly advantageous for AIDS patients who are prone to these life-threatening infections."

Source: "The Study of Spirulina: Effects on the AIDS virus, Cancer and the Immune System." The San Francisco Medical Research Foundation.

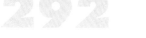

Additional Spirulina References
BOOK

Challem, J. 1981. *Spirulina*. New Canaan, CT.: Keats Publishing.

ARTICLES
Baojiang, G., et al. "Study on effect and mechanism of polysaccharides of spirulina on body immune function improvement." *Proc. of Second Asia Pacific Conf. on Algal Biotech.* Univ. of Malaysia, 1994, pp. 33–38.

Besednova, L., et al. "Immunostimulating activity of lipopolysaccharides from blue-green algae." *Zhurnal Mikrobiologii, Epidemiologii, Immunobiologii,* 56 (1979): 75–79.

Cheng-Wu, Z., T. Chao-Tsi, and Z. Zhen. "The effects of polysaccharide and phycocyanin from Spirulina platensis on peripheral blood and hematopoietic system of bone marrow in mice." *Proceedings of the Second Asia-Pacific Conference on Algal Biotechnology.* National University of Singapore, 1994, p. 58.

Hayashi, O., et al. "Class-specific influence of dietary Spirulina platensis on antibody production in mice." *Journal of Nutritional Science and Vitaminology* 44 (1998): 841–51.

Hayashi, O., T. Katoh, and Y. Okuwaki. "Enhancement of antibody production in mice by dietary Spirulina platensis." *Journal of Nutritional Science and Vitaminology* 40(1994): 431–41.

Lisheng, et al. "Inhibitive effect and mechanism of polysaccharide of spirulina on transplanted tumor cells in mice." *Marine Sciences* 5 (1991): 33–38.

Qureshi, M., J. Garlich, and M. Kidd. "Dietary Spirulina platensis enhances humeral and cell-mediated immune functions in chickens." *Immunopharmacology and Immunotoxicology* 18 (1996): 465–76.

Qureshi, M., et al. "Immune enhancement potential of Spirulina platensis in chickens." *Poultry Science.* 73 (1994): 46.

Qureshi, M., et al. "Immunomodulary effects of spirulina supplementation in chickens." In *Proc. of 44th Western Poultry Disease Conference* (1995), pp. 117–20.

Qureshi, M., and R. Ali. "Spirulina platensis exposure enhances macrophage phagocytic function in cats." *Immunopharmacology and Immunotoxicology.* 18 (1996): 457–63.

Tornabene, T., et al. "Lipid and lipopolysaccharide constituents of cyanobacterium Spirulina platensis." *Ecol Prog Serv.* 22 (1985): 121.

Blue-Green Algae
Scientific Journal References
NONTOXICITY OF BLUE-GREEN ALGAE

Algae Researcher Dr. William Barry has personally examined many blooms of the AFA strain from Klamath Lake (and other lakes, too) and has never found any toxicity. A research report produced by Rapala in *The Journal of Applied Phycology* (1993) confirmed Barry's conclusion; this report emphatically states that the AFA algae strain is not capable of producing toxins. As further testament to its safety, it should be noted that hundreds of thousands of people worldwide have consumed the AFA-strain algae with no trace of toxicity. The only time that AFA should be used cautiously is when you are extremely weak, thin, very dry with a *cold* constitution or are already pregnant.

Source: Personal communication between Gillian McKeith, PhD, and Dr. William Barry. *Miracle Superfood: Wild Blue-Green Algae,* n.d.

A taxonomic reevaluation of the paralytic shellfish toxin (saxitoxins) producing cyanobacterium *Aphanizomenon flos-aquae* LMECYA31 was done using morphology and 16S rRNA gene sequences. We found that strain LMECYA31 was incorrectly identified as Aph. flos-aquae based on (a) lack of bundle formation in trichomes, (b) shape of terminal cells in the trichomes, (c) lower similarity (97.5%) in the 16S rRNA gene sequences relative to those of Aph. flos-aquae, and (d) comparison within a phylogenetic tree of 16S rRNA gene sequences. The shape of the terminal trichome cells and the shape and size of the vegetative cell, heterocyst, and akinete in strain LMECYA31 match characters of *Aph. Issatschenkoi* (Ussachew) Proschkina-Larvernko. 16S rRNA gene sequences and phylogenetic clusters constructed from 16S rRNA gene sequences support our conclusion that strain LMECYA31 should be *Aph. issatschenkoi.* considered nontoxic, and in one situation natural populations of Aph. flos-aquae have been harvested and used as a human food supplement for over 20 years (Carmichael et al. 2000). The question of cyanotoxin production within the species *Aph. flos-aquae* deserves closer attention, and a good beginning is the taxonomic reevaluation of existing cyanotoxin producing strains that have been identified as Aph. flos-aquae. Previously we found that the PST-producing Aphanizomenon strain NH-5 was improperly identified as *Aph. flos-aquae* based on trichome shape plus 16S rRNA gene sequences (Li et al. 2000). Then Pereira et al. (2000) reported PSTs in Aph. flos-aquae strain LMECYA31 isolated from the Montargil Reservoir, Portugal. However, micrographs and descriptions in this article showed strain LMECYA31 to have elongated hyaline apical cells, a character typical of *Aph. Issatschenkoi.*

Source: Renhui, L., W. Wayne, and P. Carmichael. "Morphological and 16S rRNDA gene evidence for reclassification of the paralytic shellfish toxin producing Aphanizomenon flos-aquae LMECYA31 as Aphanizomenon Issatschenkoi (Cyanophyceae)." *J. Phycol.* 39 (2003): 814–18.

VITAMINS OF BLUE-GREEN ALGAE

The vitamin composition of blue-green algae is far superior to any multivitamin supplement pills. In a recent study at Yale New Haven Hospital, 257 brands of multivitamin supplement pills were evaluated. The study concluded that 80 percent of the vitamin pills were inadequate, incomplete, or imbalanced. With wild-blue green algae, the composition and balance of vitamins is in perfect harmony with human biochemistry for maximum utilization.

Source: Bell, L. S., and M. J. Fairchild. *American Dietetic Association.* 87 (1987): 341.

PHYCOCYANIN IN BLUE-GREEN ALGAE

Phycocyanin is the pigment that gives wild blue-green algae its blue hue; it is a protein that has been shown to inhibit the formation of cancer colonies. These various pigments operate in the body with the human pigment bilirubin to keep the liver functioning at optimum capacity, and aid in the digestion of amino acids. Phycocyanin helps draw together amino acids for neurotransmitter formation, which may increase mental capacity.

Source: Troxler, R., and B. Saffer. "Algae Derived Phycocyanin." Harvard School of Dental Medicine, Ass. Dental Research General Session Paper, 1987.

ANTI-INFLAMMATORY PROPERTIES OF PHYCOCYANIN

Phycocyanin has been shown to have strong antioxidant and anti-inflammatory properties. In various animal models of inflammation, phycocyanin was shown to reduce or prevent inflammation.

Sources: Romay, et al. "Antioxidant and anti-inflammatory properties of C-phycocyanin from blue-green algae." *Inflamm Res.* 47 (1998): 36–41.

Romay, et al. "Further studies on anti-inflammatory activity of phycocyanin in some animal models of inflammation." *Inflamm Res.* 47 (1998): 334–8.

IMPROVEMENT OF THE IMMUNE SYSTEM WITH BLUE-GREEN ALGAE

It is the high concentration of beta-carotene that activates the thymus gland; the thymus gland can then control the immune system effectively. Beta-carotene greatly enhances the immune system and may inhibit the development of cancer cells. The beta-carotene content within wild blue-green algae is extraordinarily high.

Source: Seifter, E., G. Rettura, J. Seiter, et al. "Thymotropic action of Vitamin A." *Fed. Proc.* 32 (1973): 947.

Researchers have discovered that a bacterial protein known to reduce the ability of the human immunodeficiency virus (HIV) to infect cells also inhibits infection by the Ebola virus. The antiviral protein, from blue-green algae, known as cyanovirin-N (CV-N), can extend the survival time of Ebola-infected mice, researchers from the National Cancer Institute's Molecular Targets Discovery Program report in a study published in *Antiviral Research.*

The study, done in collaboration with researchers from the U.S. Army Medical Research Institute of Infectious Diseases, the Centers for Disease Control and Prevention, and the National Institute of Diabetes and Digestive and Kidney Diseases, provides important insights into the process of Ebola infection. There is currently no treatment for Ebola infection, which causes severe and often fatal hemorrhagic fever.

Source: Barriento, L. G., et al. "Cyanovirin-N binds to the viral surface glycoprotein GP1, 2 and inhibits infectivity of Ebola virus." *Antiviral Res.* 58 (2003): 47–56.

Additional Source

http://www.appliedhealth.com/bga_biomodulator_report.html

Jensen, Gitte S., Donald I. Ginsberg, and Christian Drapeau. "Blue-Green Algae as an Immuno-Enhancer and Biomodulator." This web site article reviews the

scientific evidence for the immuno-modulatory effects of blue-green algae and some of the demonstrated effects of blue-green algae on health and disease.

SKIN CONDITIONS

My program: Gradual build-up to 3 heaping tablespoons of wild blue-green algae powder everyday (approximately 6 grams). Wild blue-green algae is rich in GLA, an essential omega-6 fatty acid that can often help to heal a faulty fat metabolism (a root cause of many skin problems). The high chlorophyll content of the algae helped to purify the blood of the toxins that cause skin eruptions. The vitality of one's skin is often related to the condition of the lungs, kidneys, or liver. For example, if your kidneys are congested, it is likely that your skin will appear lifeless, or worse. As a health practitioner, poor skin is a "red flag" for me to check the status of kidneys, lungs, or liver. When these organs are overburdened, toxins may secrete through the skin. Molecular properties of wild blue-green algae can protect and restore the liver and kidneys by clearing out the toxins.

Source: McKeith, Gillian. *Miracle Superfood: Wild Blue-Green Algae.* Los Angeles: Keats Publishing, 1999.

CHLOROPHYLL INFORMATION OF BLUE-GREEN ALGAE

Scientific research as well as popular medicine has produced evidence of the healing and anti-cancer properties of chlorophyll. For example, recent studies have reported that chlorophyllin, a water-soluble form of chlorophyll, protects against certain forms of liver cancer at a concentration similar to what is found in green leafy vegetables.

Sources: Breinholt, et al. "Dietary chlorophyllin is a potent inhibitor of aflatoxin B1 hepatocarcino-genesis in Rainbow trout." *J. Cancer Res.* 55 (1995): 57–62.

Hernaez, et al. "Effects of tea and chlorophyllin on the mutagenicity of N-hydroxy-IQ: studies of enzyme inhibition, molecular complex formation, and degradation/ scavenging of the active metabolites." *Environ Mol Mutagen.* 30 (1997): 468–74.

Negishi, et al. "Antigenotoxic activity of natural chlorophylls." *Mutat Res.* 376 (1997): 97–100.

Park, S. "Chemopreventive activity of chlorophyllin against mouse skin carcinogenesis by benzo[a]pyrene and bezo[a]pyrene-7,8-dihydrodiol-9,10-epoxide." *Cancer Lett.* 102 (1996): 143–9.

POLYUNSATURATED OMEGA-3 FATTY ACIDS IN AFA

Dietary essential fatty acids, especially omega-3 essential fatty acids, have been shown to be beneficial to the immune, cardiovascular, and nervous systems. It is interesting to note that nearly 50 percent of the lipid content of dried AFA is composed of omega-3 essential fatty acids (mostly alpha-linolenic acid).

The average North American diet is known to be lacking in omega-3 fatty acids. Such deficiency is increasingly linked to cardiovascular diseases, immunosuppression, arthritis, mental problems, and skin problems.

In addition, omega-3 fatty acids were shown to prevent platelet aggregation and to lower cholesterol. Consumption of essential fatty acids, mostly omega-3, was also shown to inhibit many forms of cancer, namely breast, prostate, pancreatic, and colon. There is also evidence that omega-3 fatty acids may help in neuropathic conditions associated with diabetes.

Sources: Bierve, K. S., O. L. Btekke, K. J. Fougner, and K. Midthiell. "Omega-3 and omega-6 fatty acids in serum lipids and their relationship to human disease." In *Dietary w3 and w6 Fatty Acids: Biological Effects and Nutritional Essentiality,* ed. C. Galli and A. P. Simopoulos. New York: Plenum, 1989, pp. 241–252.

Catalan, J., et al. "Cognitive deficits in docosahexaenoic acid-deficient rats." *Behav Neurosci.* 116 (2002): 1022–31.

DeWille, et al. "Effects of essential fatty acid deficiency and various levels of dietary polyunsaturated fatty acids, on humeral immunity in mice." *J Nutr.* 109 (1979): 1018–27.

Hibblen and Salem. "Dietary polyunsaturated fatty acids and depression: when cholesterol does not satisfy." *Am J Clin Nutr.* 62 (1995): 1–9.

Galli and Simpoulos. "Dietary omega-3 and omega-6 fatty acids: Biological effects and nutritional essentiality." *NATO ASI Series: Life Sciences,* vol. 171 (New York: Plenum Press, 1989), p. 452.

Jamal, G. A., H. Carmichael, and A. I. Weir. "Gamma-linolenic acid in diabetic neuropathy." *Lancet* 8489 (1986): 1098.

Houtsmuller, A. J., J. van Hal-Ferwerda, K. J. Zahn, and H. E. Henkes. "Favorable influences of Linoleic acid on the progression of diabetic micro- and macroangiopathy in adult onset diabetes mellitus." *Prog. Lip. Res.* 20 (1981): 377.

Kremer, et al. "Different doses of fish-oil fatty acid ingestion in active rheumatoid arthritis: a prospective study of clinical and immunological parameters." In: *Dietary Omega-3 and Omega-6 Fatty Acids: Biological Effects and Nutritional Effects and Nutritional Essentiality,* ed. C. Galli and A. P. Simopoulos. New York: Plenum, 1989, pp. 343–50.

Kremer, et al. "Fish-oil fatty acid supplementation in active rheumatoid arthritis. A double-blind controlled, crossover study." *Ann. Intern. Med.* 106 (1987): 497–503.

Nordoy, A., and T. Simonsen. "Dietary n-3 fatty acids, experimental thrombosis and coronary heart disease in man." In: *Proceedings of the AOCS short course on polyunsaturated fatty acids and eicosanoids,* ed. W. E. M. Lands. Biloxi, MS: American Oil Chemists Society, 1987, pp. 25–34.

Karmali, R. A. "Dietary Omega-3 and Omega-6 fatty acids in cancer." In: *Dietary Omega-3 and Omega-6 Fatty Acids: Biological Effects and Nutritional Effects and Nutritional Essentiality,* ed. C. Galli and A. P. Simopoulos. New York: Plenum, 1989, pp. 351-360.

Lagarde, M., M. Cropset, M., and M. Hariarine. "In vitro studies on docosahexaenoic acid in human platelets." In: *Dietary Omega-3 and Omega-6 Fatty Acids: Biological Effects and Nutritional Effects and Nutritional Essentiality,* ed. C. Galli and A. P. Simopoulos. New York: Plenum, 1989, pp. 91–96.

Siess, W., B. Scherer, B. Bohlig, P. Roth, I. Kurzmann, and P. C. Weber. 1980. "Platelet-membrane fatty acids, platelet aggregation, and thromboxane formation during a mackerel diet." *Lancet* 8166 (1980): 441–4.

Spielman, et al. "Biochemical and bioclinical aspects of blackcurrant seed oil: omega-3/omega-6 balanced oil." In: *Dietary Omega-3 and Omega-6 Fatty Acids: Biological Effects and Nutritional Effects and Nutritional Essentiality,* ed. C. Galli and A. P. Simopoulos. New York: Plenum, 1989, pp. 309–22.

Stevens, et al. "Essential Fatty acid metabolism in boys with attention-deficit hyperactivity disorder." *Am J Clin Nutr.* 62 (1995): 761–768.

Sugano, M., T. Ide, T. Ishida, and K. Yoshida. "Hypocholesterolemic effect of gamma-linolenic acid as evening primrose oil in rats." *Ann Nutr Metab.* 30 (1986): 289–99.

Wargovich, M. J. "Experimental evidence for cancer preventative elements in foods." *Cancer Letter* 114 (1997): 11–17.

Wood, et al. "Linoleic and eicosapentaenoic acids in adipose tissue and platelets and risk of coronary heart disease." *Lancet* (1987): 177–83.

Wright, S., and J. L. Burton. "Oral evening primrose seed oil improves atopic eczema." *Lancet* 8308 (1982): 1120–1122.

THE STIMULATING EFFECTS OF AFA ON NATURAL KILLER CELLS

Natural killer cells, a types of lymphocyte, are a part of the immune system and are mainly responsible for the detection and destruction of cancerous and virally infected cells in the body. In a double-blind crossover study, the immediate effect of AFA on natural killer (NK) cells was evaluated on 21 normal, healthy volunteers. Within two hours, the ingestion of AFA resulted in a significant decrease (40 percent) of NK cells in the blood. This data was interpreted to signify the migration of NK cells from the blood to the tissue, promoting immune patrolling in the tissues. Close analysis of the data revealed that this effect was barely detectable the first time individuals consumed AFA. However, after a few weeks of daily consumption of AFA, migration increased and had its maximum effect. The study shows that the benefits on the immune system are not cumulative, but come with regular daily consumption.

Source: Jensen, et al. "Consumption of *Aphanizomenon flos aquae* has rapid effects on the circulation and function of immune cells in humans." *JANA* 2 (2000): 50–58.

DEPRESSION

It was discovered nearly two decades ago that the amount of PEA in the brains of depressed patients was less than that of normal individuals and that PEA given orally to individuals suffering from depression was able to reverse the depressive condition.

Sources: Sabelli, et al. "Urinary phenyl acetate: a diagnostic test for depression?" *Science* 4602 (1983): 1187–8.

Sabelli, et al. "Sustained antidepressant effect of PeA replacement." *J Neuropsychiatry Clin Neurosci.* 8 (1996): 168–71.

Sandler, et al. "Decreased cerebrospinal fluid concentration of free phenylacetic acid in depressive illness." *Clin Chim Acta.* 93 (1979): 169–71.

ATTENTION DEFICIT DISORDER

PEA is synthesized in the brain from the two amino acids phenylalanine and

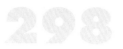

tyrosine. It is degraded by the enzyme monoamine oxilase (MAO) into pheny-lacetic acid (PAA), which is eliminated in the urine. Both PEA and PAA were found to be decreased in the urine of patients suffering from depression and ADD. The PEA precursors phenylalanine and tyrosine were also both decreased in the plasma of children suffering from ADD.

Source: Baker, et al. "Phenylethylaminergic mechanisms in attention-deficit disorder." *Biol Psychiatry* 29 (1991): 15–22.

One particular study of AFA blue-green algae is especially enlightening. It involved 109 children with an average age of 9 years, (55 girls and 54 boys) who were tak-ing blue-green algae and whose parents responded to an article placed in two national magazines across the United States. Parents filled out a detailed stan-dardized questionnaire that inquired about academic, medical, and behavioral histories of their children. At the end of the ten-week study, parents were asked to fill out another standardized questionnaire regarding improvement. Specifi-cally, parents reported "significant improvement in the ability to focus, follow directions, and concentrate ... fewer symptoms of anxiety and depression and behavior withdrawal." Teachers involved in the study also reported "an improve-ment in the ability to focus and concentrate...a reduction in aggressive and acting out behaviors." Thus, the results of this study indicate that "significant positive changes in children were evident across a wide range of behaviors . . . [and] that all children might increase their ability to concentrate and focus as AFA blue-green algae is added to their diet."

Source: C. J. Jarratt, M. D. Jewett, S. Peters, and E. Tragash. *The Children and Algae Report.* Center For Family Wellness Study, 1995.

A study conducted by the University of Central America in 1995 investigated the effects of about 1 gram of AFA blue-green algae on academic performances as well as overall health status. They monitored a group of 111 children for six months who were taking AFA blue-green algae and compared their outcomes to a control group with the same number of children. For the children taking the AFA blue-green algae, marked improvement was noted in class participation and overall ability to focus on given tasks.

Source: Seveilla, I., Aguirre, N. 1995. "Study of the effects of Super Blue Green Algae™ on the nutritional status and school performance of first, second, and third grade children attending the Monsenor Velez School in Nandaime, Nicaragua." Cell Tech.

AFA STIMULATED STEM CELL MOBILIZATION

Studies were conducted to investigate whether stem cells injected intravascularly or endogenously released from the bone marrow could cross the blood-brain bar-rier, migrate, then differentiate into brain cells. Bone marrow stem cells, along with monocytes and macrophages, were shown to have the ability to cross the blood-brain barrier and reach the brain.

Sources: Hickey, W. F. "Leukocyte traffic in the central nervous system: the participants and their roles." *Semin Immunol.* 11 (1999): 125–37.

Knopf, et al. "Antigen-dependant intrathecal antibody synthesis in the normal rat brain: tissue entry and local retention of antigen-specific B cells." *J. Immunol.* 161 (1998): 692–701.

Mezey, et al. "Turning blood into brain cells bearing neuronal antigens generated in vivo from bone marrow." *Science* 290 (2000): 1779–1782.

Williams and Hickey. "Traffic of hematogenous cells through the central nervous system." *Curr. Top. Microbiol. Immunol.* 202 (1995): 221–245.

Based on information produced by various scientific teams, Jensen et al recently proposed the "Stem Cell Theory of Healing, Regeneration, and Repair." This breakthrough theory suggests that bone marrow stem cells leave the bone marrow and travel throughout the body, providing for healing and regeneration of damaged organs during the entire lifetime of an individual. In other words, adult bone marrow stem cells may be one of the natural mechanisms that the human body utilizes for healing, regeneration, and repair.

Source: Jensen and Drapeau. 2002. "The use of *in situ* bone-marrow stem cells for the treatment of various degenerative disease." *Med Hypothesis.* 59 (2002): 422–428.

STIMULATING IMMUNE CELL MIGRATION

Natural killer (NK) cells are known scavengers of virally infected cancer cells. They destroy cells that are altered either due to viral infection or malignant transformation. They work by inducing the affected cell to undergo programmed cell death. Although NK cells are normally measured in the blood, it is in the tissues that they perform immune surveillance and eliminate virally infected or cancerous cells.

Many substances are known to improve the activity of NK cells, such as green tea and ginkgo biloba. But until this recent finding on AFA, no natural substance was known to stimulate natural killer cells to migrate into the tissues to search and destroy "sick" cells.

This research suggests that eating AFA daily may stimulate the immune system to help prevent cancer as well as illness associated with viral infections. The anticancer properties of AFA have already been established by its ability to prevent cancer in the Ames test.

Source: Lahitova, et al. "Antimutagenic properties of fresh water blue-green algae." *Folia Microbiol.* 39 (1994): 301–303.

SUMMARY OF SCIENTIFIC RESEARCH ON AFA

A thorough review of AFA's empirically reported benefits was performed by a team of scientists affiliated with the University of Illinois. The team was composed of one board-certified forensic examiner and microbiologist, one surgeon, and three physicians.

More than 200 cases that met the stringent criteria were included in this retrospective study. The study concluded that AFA seems effective in the treatment of various viral infections, chronic fatigue, Attention Deficit Disorder, depression,

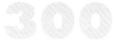
inflammatory diseases, and fibromyalgia. The study strongly suggests that AFA acts on the immune and nervous systems and prevents the process of inflammation.

Source: Krylov, et al. Retrospective epidemiological study using medical records to determine which diseases are improved by Aphanizomenon flos-aquae, submitted (2002).

Additional AFA Blue-Green Algae References

BOOKS

Drapeau, C. *Primordial Food: Aphanizomenon flos-aquae.* Asheville, NC: Unity International, 2003.

McKeith, Gillian. *Miracle Superfood: Wild Blue-Green Algae.* Los Angeles: Keats Publishing, 1999.

Price, Weston. *Nutrition and Physical Degeneration.* San Diego: Price-Pottenger Nutrition Foundation, 2008.

WEB SITES

http://www.e3live.com

Marine Phytoplankton

Scientific Journal References

NASA STUDIES ON CLOUD FORMATION

NASA-funded research has confirmed an old theory that marine phytoplankton can indirectly create clouds that block some of the sun's harmful rays. The study was conducted by Dierdre Toole of the Woods Hole Oceanographic Institution (WHOI) and David Siegel of the University of California, Santa Barbara (UCSB).

The study found that in the summer months when the sun beats down on the top layer of ocean where plankton live, harmful rays in the form of ultraviolet (UV) radiation bother the little plants. UV light also gives sunburn to humans.

When plankton are bothered, or stressed by UV light, their chemistry changes.

The plankton try to protect themselves by producing a sulfur compound called DMSP, which some scientists believe helps strengthen the plankton's cell walls. This chemical gets broken down in the water by bacteria, and changes into another substance called DMS.

DMS then evaporates from the ocean into the air, where it breaks down again to form tiny dust-like particles. These tiny particles are just the right size for large water droplets to condense on, which is the beginning of how clouds are formed. So, indirectly, marine phytoplankton help create clouds, and clouds mean that less direct light reaches the ocean surface. This relieves the stress put on plankton by the sun's harmful UV rays.

Source: http://www.nasa.gov/vision/earth/environment/0702_planktoncloud.html

HURRICANE WINDS CARRIED OCEAN SALT AND PLANKTON FAR INLAND

Researchers found surprising evidence of sea salt and frozen plankton in high, cold, cirrus clouds, the remnants of Hurricane Nora, over the U.S. plains states. Although the 1997 hurricane was a strong eastern Pacific storm, her high ice-crystal clouds extended many miles inland, carrying ocean phenomena deep into the U.S. heartland.

Kenneth Sassen of the University of Utah, Salt Lake City, and University of Alaska Fairbanks; W. Patrick Arnott of the Desert Research Institute (DRI) in Reno, Nevada; and David O. Starr of NASA's Goddard Space Flight Center, Greenbelt, Maryland, co-authored a paper about Hurricane Nora's far-reaching effects. The paper was published in the April 1, 2003, issue of the *American Meteorological Society's Journal of Atmospheric Sciences.*

Scientists were surprised to find what appeared to be frozen plankton in some cirrus crystals collected by research aircraft over Oklahoma, far from the Pacific Ocean. This was the first time examples of microscopic marine life, like plankton, were seen as "nuclei" of ice crystals in the cirrus clouds of a hurricane.

PLANKTON MAY INFLUENCE CLIMATE CHANGE SAYS UCSB SCIENTIST

Plankton appear to play a major role in regulating the global climate system, according to new research.

David Siegel, professor of geography at the University of California, Santa Barbara, and director of the Institute for Computational Earth System Science, made the discovery with his former PhD student Dierdre Toole, who is now based at Woods Hole Oceanographic Institute.

In an article in the May 6 issue of the journal *Geophysical Research Letters,* the scientists explain their research in the Sargasso Sea, approximately 50 miles southeast of the island of Bermuda. Siegel's research group has been making observations at this location since 1992.

Phytoplankton are tiny, single-celled floating plants. They inhabit the upper layers of any natural body of water where there is enough light to support photosynthetic growth. They are the base of the ocean's food web, and their production helps to regulate the global carbon cycle. They also contribute to the global cycling of many other compounds with climate implications.

One of these compounds is a volatile organic sulfur gas called dimethyl sulfide or DMS. Scientists had previously theorized that DMS is part of a climate feedback mechanism, but until now there had been no observational evidence illustrating how reduced sunlight actually leads to the decreased ocean production of DMS. This is the breakthrough in Toole and Siegel's research. They describe how the cycle begins when the ocean gives off DMS to the lower atmosphere. In the air, DMS breaks down into a variety of sulfur compounds that act as cloud-condensing nuclei, leading to increased cloudiness. With more clouds, less sunlight reaches the Earth and the biological processes that produce DMS are reduced.

According to their research, it appears that phytoplankton produce organic sulfur compounds (DMSP, DMS, DMSO) as a chemical defense from the damaging effects of ultraviolet radiation and other environmental stresses, in much the same way as our bodies use vitamins E and C to flush out molecules that cause cellular damage.

DMSO and its metabolite methyl-sulfonyl-methane (MSM) are known potent antioxidants, are also effective in human nutrition, and protect against human skin against ultraviolet radiation damage.

Siegel and Toole found that ultraviolet radiation explained almost 90 percent of the variability in the biological production of DMS. They showed that summertime DMS production is "enormous," and that the entire upper layer of DMS content is replaced in just a few days. This demonstrates a tight link between DMS and solar fluxes.

"The significance of this work is that it provides, for the first time, observational evidence showing that the DMS-antioxidant mechanism closes the DMS-climate feedback loop," said Siegel. "The implications are huge. Now we know that phytoplankton respond dramatically to UV radiation stresses, and that this response is incredibly rapid, literally just days."

Sources: http://earthobservatory.nasa.gov///Newsroom/MediaAlerts/2002/200204
258802.html

http://phytoplankton.gsfc.nasa.gov/

http://www.mos.org/oceans/life/webs.html

http://en.wikipedia.org/wiki/Diatom

SHEWANELLA PHYTOPLANKTON AND DMSO

The incredible diversity of microbes from hydrothermal vent systems to subglacial Antarctic lake environments is a testament to metabolic innovation. Microbes are found essentially anywhere they can take advantage of chemical gradients to generate energy by using a diverse repertoire of biochemical tools.

Shewanella species have been isolated from many aquatic environments. The cosmopolitan nature of this species is likely because of their incredible respiratory versatility. Various *Shewanella* strains are reported to use approximately 20 different terminal electron acceptors for respiration. One of these compounds, dimethyl sulfoxide (DMSO), is found in significant concentrations throughout aquatic environments, sometimes representing the most abundant methylated sulfur compound present. DMSO can be produced from the photochemical oxidation of dimethyl sulfide (DMS), but the major source appears to be marine phytoplankton. Another potential source is bacterial oxidation of DMS to DMSO, although it is unclear whether this process is significant in marine systems. DMS can be produced both from the reduction of DMSO and from the enzymatic breakdown of dimethylsulfoniopropionate (DMSP). DMSP, in turn, is synthesized by a variety of marine phytoplankton as an osmoregulator, cryoprotectant, and radical scavenger. Globally, the DMSP/DMS/DMSO cycle is important with respect to climate, because DMS is an anti-greenhouse gas, directly impacting cloud formation where it is produced in significant quantities.

Despite this importance, very little is understood regarding how aquatic bacteria produce DMS through respiration of DMSO. Although commonly thought to be a soluble compound, DMSO can be associated with particulate material in marine systems.

Here we demonstrate that the DMSO reductase in *Shewanella oneidensis* is localized to the outside of the cell. The localization of this enzyme suggests that DMSO acquisition may be difficult in the environments *Shewanella* inhabits, perhaps because of its physical inaccessibility or the challenge of transporting it. We discuss how utilization of this compound by *Shewanella* might influence the geochemical cycling of sulfur in aquatic systems.

Shewanella species are renowned for their respiratory versatility, including their ability to respire poorly soluble substrates by using enzymatic machinery that is localized to the outside of the cell. This study shows that DMSO respiration is an extracellular respiratory process through the analysis of mutants defective in type II secretion, which is required for transporting proteins to the outer membrane in *Shewanella*. Moreover, immunogold labeling of DMSO reductase subunits reveals that they reside on the outer leaflet of the outer membrane under anaerobic conditions. The extracellular localization of the DMSO reductase in *S. oneidensis* suggests these organisms may perceive DMSO in the environment as an insoluble compound.

Source: http://www.pubmedcentral.nih.gov/articlerender.fcgi?artid=1450229
"Extracellular respiration of dimethyl sulfoxide by *Shewanella oneidensis* strain MR-1"
Jeffrey A. Gralnick, Hojatollah Vali, Douglas P. Lies, and Dianne K. Newman
(2005).

COMPLEXITY OF EPA AND DHA FROM PHYTOPLANKTON IN REGULATING MARINE ECOSYSTEMS

Summary: Long-chain n-3 polyunsaturated fatty acids (LCn-3 PUFAs) such as EPA and DHA are important biomolecules regulating production in marine ecosystems. This study examined how the interaction at the phytoplankton-zooplankton interface affected the transfer of LCn-3 PUFAs to higher trophic levels. Heterotrophic dinoflagellates contained higher levels of EPA and DHA than their algal prey, suggesting heterotrophic dinoflagellates enhanced the nutritional value of poor quality algae and subsequent transfer to the next trophic level. Formation of EPA and DHA in the dinoflagellates appears to be achieved by the elongation and desaturation of shorter fatty acid chains rather than through de novo synthesis.

Fatty acid content in the copepod *Acartia tonsa* resembled the fatty acid signature of its prey, further supporting the idea that heterotrophs depend on their diet to obtain these nutrients, and their nutritional value is subject to the type of food consumed. Transfer of DHA to *A. tonsa,* was improved by feeding on a heterotrophic dinoflagellate grown on a poor quality algae, versus feeding on the algae itself. Thus omnivorous copepods may compensate dietary deficiencies by feeding on a variety of prey items.

The presence of EPA and DHA can be used as a proxy for the nutritional value of copepods. *A. tonsa* fed nutritiously poor algae also affected the fatty acid content of its predator. *Pseudopleuronectes americanus* fed low-quality copepods, had lower levels of EPA and DHA than those fed copepods with higher levels of these fatty acids. However, content of these fatty acids did not have a direct effect on the growth rate of the fish. The finding herein does not support consumption of LCn-3 PUFAs as important factors regulating growth in juvenile fish. These results, albeit discouraging, are by no means comprehensive in elucidating the role of n-3 PUFAs for fish health. It is possible that due to food limitation, the effect of food quality was confounded.

Field collected data in a nursery ground for juvenile *P. americanus* showed that the quantity of EPA and DHA in the prey for the fish at the time of sampling was low. The low availability of these fatty acids in the plankton suggests this estuary is at times suboptimal for the growth and development of *P. americanus.* EPA and DHA are critical for *P. americanus* growth; however, the low availability of LCn-3 PUFAs does not by itself explain differences in growth rates. It is clear that further field studies should combine physical, biological, and chemical factors in order to evaluate the nutritional status of the nursery ground.

Source: Veloza, Adriana J. "Transfer of Essential Fatty Acids by Marine Phytoplankton." A Thesis Presented to The Faculty of the School of Marine Science (The College of William and Mary), 2005.

Additional Marine Phytoplankton Reference

ARTICLE

Mike Adams. August 14, 2008. "Marine Phytoplankton is Next Revolutionary Superfood for Disease Prevention and Extraordinary Health." http://www.naturalnews.com/023853.html

Aloe Vera

Scientific Journal References

BOOSTING ANTIOXIDANT ACTIVITY

Antioxidants, particularly glutathione, are in short supply in CFS, fibromyalgia, and Gulf War syndrome; an increase in free-radical generation often occurs as well. In human studies, cordyceps extracts and Cs-4 have been shown to scavenge free radicals and so may be beneficial. And in animal and in vitro studies, *aloe vera* extracts, polysaccharide K, and reishi mushroom have been potent stimulators of glutathione, which destroys free radicals.

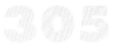

Sources: Kim, H. S., S. Kacew, and B. M. Lee. "In vitro chemopreventive effects of plant polysaccharides (*Aloe barbadensis, Lentinus Edodes, Ganoderma lucidum,* and *Coriolus versicolor.*)" *Carcinogenesis* 20 (1999): 1637–40.

Pang, Z. J., Y. Chen, M. Zhou, and J. Wan. "Effect of polysaccharide krestin on glutathione peroxidase gene expression in mouse peritoneal macrophages." *Br J Biomed Sci.* 57 (2000): 130–36.

Richards, R. S., T. K. Roberts, R. H. Dustan, et al. "Free radicals in chronic fatigue syndrome: cause or effect?" *Redox Rep.* 5 (2000): 146–147.

Sabeh, F., T. Wright, and S. J. Norton. "Purification and characterization of a glutathione peroxidase from the aloe vera plant." *Enzyme Protein.* 47 (1993): 92–98.

Zhu, J. S., G. M. Halpern, and K. Jones. "The scientific rediscovery of an ancient Chinese herbal medicine: Cordyceps sinensis (Part I)." *J Altern Complement Med.* 4 (1998): 295.

RHEUMATOID ARTHRITIS

We know more about aloe's effects on arthritis, at least in animals. When researchers treated arthritic rats with *aloe vera,* the result was a 50 percent decrease in inflammation. Mast cells, activated in allergic and autoimmune phenomena, also decreased by 48 percent. In addition, the aloe stimulated an increase in fibroblasts, which grow and repair the tissue. Other studies indicate that aloe extracts markedly inhibit induced arthritis, edema, and inflammation in rodents.

Sources: Davis, R. H., and N. P. Maro. "Aloe vera and gibberellin. Anti-inflammatory activity in diabetes." *J Am Podiatr Med Assoc.* 79 (1989): 24–26.

Davis, R. H., G. J. Stewart, and P. J. Bregman. "Aloe vera and the inflamed synovial pouch model." *J Am Podiatr Med Assoc.* 82 (1992): 140–48.

Saito, H., T. Ishiguro, K. Imanishi, and I. Suzuki. "Pharmacological studies on plant lectin aloctin A. II. Inhibitory effect of aloctin A on experimental models of inflammation in rats." *Jpn J Pharmacol.* 32 (1982): 139–42.

JUVENILE DIABETES

In 1981, researchers examined the mucous from the bowels of ten patients with Crohn's disease and compared it with that of normal controls. More than half of the normal colons registered eight or more monosaccharides, whereas about a quarter of those with ulcerative colitis and Crohn's registered eight or more of these sugars. What may help people with these disorders is *aloe vera.* In a series of human trials, acemannan from aloe improved food digestion and absorption and enhanced "good" bacterial flora in the digestive tract, by reducing yeast and pH levels. Additionally, we know that gum sugars called arabinogalactans may help those with digestive tract problems, including irritable bowel syndrome. The glyconutrients are poorly digested and ferment in the large intestine. While this sounds like something better avoided, it's actually good: the fermentation produces short-chain fatty acids, crucial for preventing and alleviating diarrhea. One of the most important of these fatty acids is called butyrate or butyric acid, a crucial metabolite for colon health.

Sources: Clamp, J. R., G. Frasier, and A. E. Read. "Study of the carbohydrate content of mucous glycoproteins from normal and diseased colons." *Clin Sci* (Colch). 61 (1981): 229–34.

Kelly, G. S. "Larch arabinogalactan: Clinical relevance of a novel immune-enhancing polysaccharide." *Altern Med Rev.* 4 (1999): 96–103.

Reynolds, T., and A. C. Dweck. "Aloe vera leaf gel: A review update." *J Ethnopharmacol.* 68 (1999): 15.

RADIATION AND GLYCONUTRIENTS

Glyconutrients, including reishi mushroom and *aloe vera,* have been found to decrease radiation sickness in animals and to help them recover faster. Animals given these glyconutrients gained weight faster and were less nauseated, and their blood counts returned to normal faster than did the counts of controls that were irradiated but did not receive glyconutrients. Topical preparations have also proved to be helpful. In one double-blind study on mice conducted at the renowned M.D. Anderson Cancer Center in Houston, Texas, a topical gel containing acemannan from aloe reduced skin reactions to radiation significantly. The glyconutrient also increased the amount of radiation required to inflict skin damage. Researchers found that the gel was most effective if applied daily for at least two weeks immediately after each radiation treatment. The scientists found that aloe didn't work if applied before irradiation or beginning one week after irradiation.

Sources: Egger, S. F., G. S. Brown, L. S. Kelsey, et al. 1996. "Hematopoietic augmentation by a beta-(1,4)-linked mannan." *Cancer Immunol Immunother.* 43 (1996): 195–205.

Hsu, H. Y., S. L. Lian, and C. C. Lin. "Radioprotective effect of Ganoderma lucidum (Leyss. Ex. Fr.) Karst after X-ray irradiation in mice." *AM J Chin Med.* 18 (1990): 61–69.

Pande, S., M. Kuymar, and A. Kumar. "Radioprotective efficacy of aloe vera leaf extract." *Pharmaceut Biol.* 36 (1998): 227–232.

Roberts, D. B., and E. L. Travis. "Acemannan-containing wound dressing gel reduces radiation-induced skin reactions in C3H mice." *Int J Radiat Oncol Biol Phys.* 32 (1995): 1047–52.

ALOE, MELATONIN, CANCER

In a study conducted in Milan, Italy, twenty-six patients with advanced solid tumors (including cancers of the breast, gastrointestinal tract, brain, and lung) who hadn't responded to traditional therapy, were treated daily with 20 milligrams of melatonin, which has been shown to induce some benefits for untreatable metastized cancer patients. Another twenty-four patients received 20 milligrams of melatonin daily plus a tincture (alcohol-based liquid) of *aloe vera,* 1 milliliter twice a day. A partial response achieved in two of the twenty-four patients treated with melatonin plus aloe, whereas none of the patients treated with melatonin alone improved. In addition, the cancer stabilized in fourteen of the aloe patients, compared with only seven of the melatonin patients.

Source: Lissoni, P., L. Giani, S. Zerbini, et al. "Biotherapy with the pineal immunomodulating hormone melatonin versus melatonin plus *aloe vera* in untreatable advanced solid neoplasms." *Nat Immun.* 16 (1998): 27–33.

STAVING OFF FAT, PRESERVING MUSCLE

Using a DEXA scan, which measures the percentage of body fat and lean tissue (it can also measure bone density), researchers studied 136 overweight people. One group was placed on weight-loss drugs and a recommended diet and exercise plan in step with their weight goal. Another group was placed on a weight-loss drug, a diet and exercise plan, as well as *aloe vera* extracts and phytochemicals (freeze-dried fruits and vegetables). The third group was placed on a diet and exercise plan, *aloe vera* and phytochemical supplements—but no weight-loss drugs.

DEXA scans were conducted at the beginning and at the end of the sixty-day study. The scientists found that those on glyconutrients and phytochemicals *consistently gained lean tissue and lost fat to a more significant degree than those on the drugs alone.*

Specifically, the drug-only group lost 0.8 percent body fat, as compared to 4 percent in the drug/supplement group and 3.5 percent in the supplement-only group. The drug-only group lost 2.9 pounds of muscle, whereas the drug supplement group gained 2.4 pounds of muscle and the supplement-only group *gained* nearly 4 pounds of muscle. The two groups that took weight-loss drugs each lost about 8.5 pounds, whereas the supplement group lost only 4 pounds but keep in mind that the supplement-only group gained more muscle than the other two groups, and muscle is denser and weighs more than fat. That's why muscular people may weigh more but look slimmer than their flabby counterparts.

How much weight loss was attributable to the *aloe vera* and how much to phytochemicals in this study isn't known, though animal studies confirm that glyconutrients alone aid in weight loss. In one study, scientists at the Kobe Pharmaceutical University in Japan fed ten young rats with high cholesterol and triglyceride levels a high-fat diet laced with maitake powder. The ten controls received the high-fat feed without the mushroom powder. After twenty-four days, while both groups had put on weight, the controls had put on considerably more. As an added maitake bonus, the maitake rats registered significantly lower triglyceride and total cholesterol levels than the controls at the end of the study.

Sources: Kaats, G. R., S. C. Keith, H. A. Croft, et al. "Dietary supplements and a behavior modification plan improve the safety and efficacy of pharmacotherapy." *Adv Ther.* 15 (1998): 167–179.

Kubo, K., and H. Nanba. "The effect of maitake mushrooms on liver and serum lipids." *Altern Ther.* 2 (1996): 62–66.

SUN DAMAGE

Sunscreen does nothing to reverse skin damage once the damage is done. And if the damage is severe enough, it may induce suppression of Langerhans cells, located in the skin's epidermis, the outer layer of skin. This suppression results in reduced immunity in the skin, which may precede malignancy. Langerhans cells, a kind of macrophage, coordinate the actions of the immune system, orchestrating skin healing. *Aloe vera* gel has been shown to prevent the suppression of these cells in mice, thereby preventing ultraviolet-induced immune suppression in the skin. In animals, aloe's ability to prevent skin damage from the sun and from radiation treatment for cancer has been documented extensively. In 1994, a research team at M.D. Anderson Cancer Center in Houston, Texas, found that mice exposed to UVB showed diminished immune response, with up to 90 percent less macrophage activity than in controls. Exposure to UVB can suppress immunity not only at the skin level but also throughout the body. Applying aloe gel to the skin within twenty-four hours after exposure to ultraviolet light restored Langerhans cells and immune functioning both locally and systemically. M.D. Anderson scientists also reported that ordinary skin cells exposed to ultraviolet rays showed decreased immune response, but aloe extracts restored the immune system response to normal.

Sources: Byeon, S. W., et al. "Aloe barbadensis extracts reduce the production of interleukin-10 after exposure to ultraviolet radiation." *J Invest Dermatol.* 110 (1998): 811–17.

Lee, C. K., S. S. Han, Y. K. Mo, et al. "Prevention of ultraviolet radiation-induced suppression of accessory cell function of Langerhans cells by aloe vera gel components." *Immunopharmacology.* 37 (1997): 153–162.

——"Acemannan-containing wound dressing gel reduces radiation-induced skin reactions in C3H mice." *Int J Radiat Oncol Biol Phys.* 32 (1997): 1047–52.

Strickland, F. M., R. P. Pelley, and M. L. Kripke. "Prevention of ultraviolet radiation-induced suppression of contact and delayed hypersensitivity by Aloe barbadensis gel extract." *J Invest Dermatol.* 102 (1994): 197–204.

OTHER GLYCONUTRIENTS

Aloe and psyllium lower cholesterol, too. In a five-year controlled study of five thousand patients with angina—chest pain caused by insufficient blood flow to the heart from coronary artery disease—those participants given *aloe vera* and Isabgol husks, a psyllium fiber that contains polysaccharides, achieved a marked reduction in total serum cholesterol, serum triglycerides, and total lipids, as well as an increase in HDL. The clinical picture improved as well: frequency of angina attacks went down, and patients needed less medication, including drugs called beta-blockers, commonly used to treat heart disease. Interestingly, the patients who most benefited were diabetics. Other studies have confirmed psyllium's ability to lower LDL and decrease cholesterol absorption in men with high cholesterol.

Sources: Agarwal, O. P. "Prevention of atheromatous heart disease." *Angiology* 36 (1985): 485–92.

Everson, G. T., B. P. Daggy, C. McKinley, and J. A. Story. "Effects of psyllium hydrophilic mucilloid on LDL-cholesterol and bile acid synthesis in hypercholesterolemic men." *J Lipid Res.* 33 (1992): 1183–92.

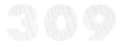
Additional Aloe Vera References

BOOKS

Mondoa, Emil I., and Mindy Kitei. *Sugars That Heal.* New York: Ballantine Books, 2002.

Skousen, Mark B. *Aloe Vera Handbook.* Summertown, TN: Healthy Living Publications, 2003.

Hemp

Interesting Hemp Facts

Hemp materials have been found in the ashen ruins of Pompeii.

The Vikings used hemp sails.

By the eighth-century the hemp papermaking techniques from China had spread to Arabia and Persia.

Around 1150 the Moors started manufacturing hemp paper in Spain.

Both the Gutenberg Bible (fifteenth century) and the King James Bible (seventeenth century) were printed on hemp paper.

In 1619, America's first hemp law was enacted at Jamestown colony "ordering" all farmers to grow hemp. Similarly, mandatory hemp cultivation laws were enacted in Massachusetts, Connecticut, and in the Chesapeake colonies into the mid-1700s.

The Declaration of Independence was written and signed on hemp paper.

The original California 49er Levi-Strauss jeans were made from hemp canvas (sail cloth) and rivets.

The original American flags, including Old Glory, were made from hemp fiber.

The parachute that saved George Bush Sr.'s life in World War II was made of hemp fiber.

Additional Hemp References

BOOKS

Erasmus, Udo. *Fats That Heal, Fats That Kill.* Canada: Alive Publishing, 2001.

Jones, K. *Nutritional and Medicinal Guide to Hemp Seed.* Canada: Rainforest Botanical Laboratory, 1995.

Suzar. *Drugs Masquerading as Foods.* Ojai, CA: A-Kar Productions, 1999.

WEB SITES

http://www.thehia.org/facts.html

http://naihc.org/hemp_information/hemp_facts.html

http://www.hempfarm.org/Papers/Hemp_Facts.html

http://www.globalhemp.com/Archives/FAQ/interesting_facts_on_hemp.html

http://www.ratical.org/renewables/plywood.html

Coconut

Scientific Journal References

MORE ON COCONUT'S MCFAS

Coconuts play a unique role in the diets of mankind because they are the source of important physiologically functional components. These physiologically functional components are found in the fat part of whole coconut, in the fat part of desiccated coconut, and in the extracted coconut oil.

Lauric acid, the major fatty acid from the fat of the coconut, has long been recognized for the unique properties that it lends to nonfood uses in the soaps and cosmetics industry. More recently, lauric acid has been recognized for its unique properties in food use, which are related to its antiviral, antibacterial, and antiprotozoal functions. Now, capric acid, another of coconut's fatty acids, has been added to the list of coconut's antimicrobial components. These fatty acids are found in the largest amounts only in traditional lauric fats, especially from coconut. Also, recently published research has shown that natural coconut fat in the diet leads to a normalization of body lipids, protects against alcohol damage to the liver, and improves the immune system's anti-inflammatory response.

Clearly, there has been increasing recognition of the health-supporting functions of the fatty acids found in coconut. Recent reports from the U.S. Food and Drug Administration requiring the labeling of trans-fatty acids will put coconut oil in a more competitive position and may help its return to use by the baking and snack-food industry, where it has continued to be recognized for its functionality. Now it can be recognized for another kind of functionality: the improvement of the health of mankind.

Source: Enig, Mary G. "The Health Benefits of Coconuts and Coconut Oil." *Nexus Magazine* 9:2 (2001).

COCONUT AGAINST SARS

Health Secretary Manuel Dayrit stirred the national adrenalin at the Senate hearing on Severe Acute Respiratory Syndrome (SARS) recently when he unveiled virgin coconut oil as a potential cure for viral epidemics.

While the senators cackled over the appellation "virgin," Dayrit was careful to mark the word "potential."

Dayrit is well aware of the potential of virgin coconut oil. His own father, Dr. Conrado Dayrit, M.D., has been successful in using virgin coconut oil since 1980 to combat the AIDS virus among AIDS patients in the San Lazaro Hospital.

The elder Dayrit is currently conducting test applications of virgin coconut oil to SARS patients in cooperation with The Research Institute for Tropical Medicine at Alabang. Medical director of the Potenciano Medical Center (formerly Polymedic), emeritus professor of pharmacology, University of the Philippines and past president of the National Academy of Science and Technology, Dayrit has been quietly at work on 14 patients ages 22 to 48 on a shoestring budget.

In the 1980s, Dayrit's was the first clinical study on coconut oil, which led to the breakthrough discovery that medium-chain fatty acids (MCFA)—lauric and capric—were effective in killing human immunodeficiency virus (HIV) in lab cultures.

Since the HIV is a lipid-coated virus as is the SARS coronavirus, there is a high probability that virgin coconut oil can produce the same effect on the latter. *Source:* Villariba, Cesar C. "Virgin Coconut Oil Being Tested On SARS Patients." *Phillipine Daily Inquirer* (May 18, 2003).

Additional Coconut References

BOOKS

Erasmus, Udo. *Fats That Heal, Fats That Kill.* Canada: Alive Publishing, 2001.
Wolfe, David. *Eating For Beauty.* Berkeley: North Atlantic Books, 2009.

WEB SITES

http://coconutboard.nic.in/tendnutr.htm
http://en.wikipedia.org/wiki/Coconut
http://www.thaifoodandtravel.com/features/cocgood.html

ARTICLE

Blackburn, G. L., et al. "A reevaluation of coconut oil's effect on serum cholesterol and atherogenesis." *Journal of the Philippine Medical Association* 65 (1989): 144–52.

Açai

The Acai Research Organization (www.acairesearch.org)

"Brazilian Berry Destroys Cancer Cells in Lab." *Journal of Agricultural and Food Chemistry.* [Filed under *Research, Health, Sciences, Agriculture* on Thursday, January 12, 2006.]

Camu Camu Berry

[The author's field notes and scientific research, now posted on many web sites across the Internet.]

Chlorella

Scientific References

"Augmentation of host defense by a unicellular green alga, Chlorella Vulgaris, to Escherichia coli infection." *Infection and Immunity* 53(1986): 267–71.

"Effect of Chlorella Vulgaris Extracts on Murine Cytomegalovirus Infections," *Nat Immun Cell Growth Regul.* 9 (1990): 121–28.

"Accelerated restoration of the leukocyte number and augmented resistance against Escherichia coli in cyclophosphamide-treated rats orally administered with a hot water extract of chlorella vulgaris." *Int. Jrnl. Immunopharmacology.* 12 (1990): 883–91.

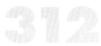

"The Effects of Chlorella Vulgaris in the protection of mice infected with Listeria monocytogenes, role of natural killer cells." *Immunopharmacology and Immunotoxicology* 21 (1999): 609–19.

Web Sites

http://www.healingdaily.com/oral-chelation/health-benefits-of-chlorella.htm
http://www.health-books.com/NaturalHealth/StrengthenYourDefenses_p39.htm
http://sunchlorella.com.au/key_benefits_wakasa.htm
http://www.ace-nutrition.com/chlorella-nutritional-analysis.html
http://www.juicing.com/sunchlorella.htm
http://www.diagnose-me.com/treat/T63897.html

Incan Berries

[The author's field notes and scientific research, now posted on many web sites across the Internet.]

Kelp

IODINE

Elson M. Haas, MD

http://www.howstuffworks.com/framed.htm?parent=question367.htm&url=http://www.healthy.net/library/books/haas/minerals/i.htm

(Excerpted from *Staying Healthy with Nutrition: The Complete Guide to Diet and Nutritional Medicine*)

http://www.acu-cell.com/sni.html

Noni

Fairechild, Diana. *Noni: Aspirin of the Ancients.* Hawaii: Flyana Rhyme, 1998.

Yacon Root

[The author's field notes and scientific research, now posted on many web sites across the Internet.]

Photo Credits

Shazzie (www.shazzie.com)

Juliana Garske

Camille Perrin

David Wolfe

Christopher Wodtke (www.kirlian.com)

Spirulina images generously provided by Cyanotech Corporation (www.cyanotech.com). Used with permission.

AFA Blue-Green Algae and Klamath Lake images generously provided by David Robatcek and Klamath Algae Products (www.E3Live.com). Copyright © David Robatcek. Used with permission.

Cacao image on p. 55 © iStockphoto.com/eefauscan

Coconut image on p. 207 © iStockphoto.com/AlexMax

Coconut image on p. 208 © iStockphoto.com/AlexMax

Index

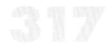

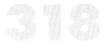

Index

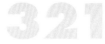

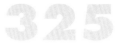

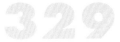

About the Author

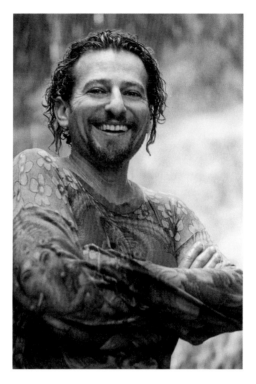

David "Avocado" Wolfe (born August 6, 1970, 11:43 a.m., near New York City) is considered by peers to be one of the world's leading authorities on nutrition. David develops and distributes some of the world's most wonderful and exotic organic food items. David was the first to bring raw and organic cacao beans/nibs (raw chocolate), goji berries, Incan berries, cacao butter, cacao powder, powdered encapsulated mangosteen, maca extract, cold-pressed coconut oil, and Sacred Chocolate™ into general distribution in North America. Known for extraordinary quality control and ethical production, these products, and many others developed by David, lead the field.

The son of two medical doctors, David brings a unique perspective on health and nutrition to the world of superfoods. He holds degrees in mechanical and environmental engineering, political science, a Juris doctor in law degree, and a master's degree in living-food nutrition. He has studied at many institutions, including Oxford University. David still participates in higher education as a professor of nutrition for Dr. Gabriel Cousens's master's degree program on live-food nutrition.

Since 1995, David has given well over a thousand health lectures and seminars in the United States, Canada, Europe, the South Pacific, Central America, and South America. As part of his action-packed schedule, David also coaches and feeds Hollywood producers and celebrities as well as some of the world's leading business people and entrepreneurs. The author of *The Sunfood Diet Success System, Naked Chocolate, Eating for Beauty,* and *Amazing Grace,* he hosts at least six health, fitness, and adventure retreats each year at various retreat centers across the world. You may view his current schedule at www.davidwolfe.com. David is the founder of and leading contributor to the Internet's leading peak performance and nutrition magazine: www.thebestdayever.com. He is also founder of the nonprofit Fruit Tree Planting Foundation (www.ftpf.org) whose goal is to plant eighteen billion fruit trees on planet Earth.

Other than his passion for nutrition, David's favorite hobbies include drumming, gardening, hiking, yoga, literature, writing, alchemy, chemistry, wild adventures, hot springs soaking, planting fruit trees, spending time with loved ones, and having The Best Day Ever!

www.davidwolfe.com
www.thebestdayever.com
www.sacredchocolate.com

To book David Wolfe on a television or radio show, for an interview, or a seminar, please contact Angela Hartman at: angelahartman333@gmail.com

Sacred Chocolate™

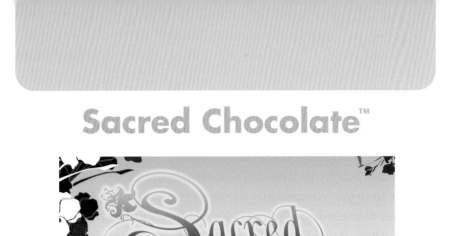

"Sacred Chocolate™ is clearly the best chocolate bar ever. Take one bite and you will know that Sacred Chocolate™ has cracked the cacao code!"

—David Wolfe

Sacred Chocolate™ is committed to bringing you the highest quality chocolate ever. From the cacao bean to each chocolate bar, Sacred Chocolate™ is infused with love, prayer, and gratitude. We honor, respect, and give thanks to all beings that make the amazing superfood known as chocolate possible. *Theobroma cacao* is the scientific name for the chocolate tree, which means the "food of God." To our Sacred Chocolate™ team, this food is a holy sacrament, an offering to the higher power, and a superfood for positive life transformation.

Our special chocolate is made over several days, the old-fashioned way: we slowly stone-grind our raw cacao beans at a low temperature. Our single, unique *aromica* variety of Ecuadorian cacao beans are never roasted, and all processes are kept below 114 degrees Fahrenheit to ensure maximum antioxidant retention and zero trans-fatty acid production. Sacred Chocolate™ has an antioxidant rating (ORAC score) three to four times higher than that of a cooked dark chocolate bar of comparable cacao content. Our ingredients are raw (unroasted) wherever possible and always certified organic and/or wild-crafted. Sacred Chocolate™ is also certified Vegan, Kosher, and Halal. Our cacao is sold above Fair Trade standards.

We never use weak cacao "filler" beans to boost cacao percentage, and we completely avoid cane sugar in all our products. Sacred Chocolate™ is extremely low in caffeine, and, like all chocolate, contains theobromine, which is much superior to caffeine, since theobromine has cardiovascular and lung-healing properties. Theobromine does not affect the central nervous system or constrict blood vessels. For those who want to reduce their coffee consumption, Sacred Chocolate™ is the healthiest alternative. Theobromine dilates blood vessels and relaxes smooth muscle tissue, reducing the risk of cardiovascular challenges. For nearly four decades (1890–1930), theobromine was injected into the bloodstream to revive heart attack victims.

Sacred Chocolate™ comes in the shape of a heart to symbolize that raw chocolate is good for the heart and that great love and care go into the making of Sacred Chocolate™. Theobromine also relaxes bronchial muscles in the lungs. Studies indicate that theobromine acts on the vagus nerve, which runs from the lungs to the brain. For this reason, chocolate has been found to be effective in reducing asthma symptoms. Sacred Chocolate™ is the only chocolate product in the world that includes the microbe-free skin of the cacao bean for flavor and nutritional purposes. The delicate skin adds a fruity complexity to the flavor of Sacred Chocolate™ and also adds concentrated phytonutrients, analogous to the nutrition found in the skin of most fruits and vegetables. Sacred Chocolate™ uses certifiably vegan, organic maple sugar in all sweetened recipes. The maple bouquet adds a rich complexity to the fruity *aromica* bean. Also, by using maple, old-growth forests thrive—trees are not cut down to produce it. Maple rates low with a score of fifty-five on the glycemic index, and contains manganese, zinc, and potassium, as well as antioxidants including epicatechins and quercetin.

Five percent of Sacred Chocolate™ profits are donated to the Fruit Tree Planting Foundation (ftpf.org).

Now is the best time ever to visit:
www.SacredChocolate.com

"Open the Heart . . . Discover the Magic!"

The Fruit Tree Planting Foundation
(www.ftpf.org)

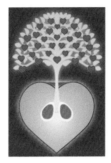

"Nothing in the world gives me more satisfaction than planting fruit trees. As I have always chosen to channel my energy and finances into environmentally friendly, sustainable, and healthy directions, I founded the nonprofit Fruit Tree Planting Foundation as a place where we could all vote with our money for a better, happier, more abundant, forested future on Earth. Please read about our foundation and decide that you want to donate your time, energy, and/or money to this worthy cause."

—David Wolfe

The Fruit Tree Planting Foundation (FTPF) is a unique nonprofit charity dedicated to planting edible, fruitful trees and plants to benefit needy populations and improve the surrounding air, soil, and water. We strategically plant orchards where the harvest will best serve the community for decades to follow, at places such as homeless shelters, drug rehab centers, low-income areas, international hunger relief sites, and animal sanctuaries. FTPF's projects benefit the environment, human health, and animal welfare—all at once!

FTPF's goal is straightforward: to collectively plant eighteen billion fruit trees for a healthy planet (approximately three for every person alive).

Fruit trees heal the environment by cleaning the air, improving soil quality, preventing erosion, creating animal habitat, sustaining valuable water sources, and providing healthy nutrition. We envision a place where one can have a summer picnic under the shade of a fruit tree, breathe the clean air it generates, listen to the songbirds it attracts, and not have to bring anything other than an appetite for the healthy fruits growing overhead. A world where one can take a walk in the park during a lunch break, pick and eat a variety of delicious fruits, plant the seeds so others can eventually do the same, and provide an alternative to buying environmentally destructive, illness-causing, chemically laden products.

FTPF has planted thousands of fruit trees all over the world and provided advice and training for others to do so as well. We have launched a series of exciting new programs, and we need your help! Your tax-deductible charitable investment will help us realize our dream of a sustainable planet for generations to come. If you find you are interested in donating, please send a check or money order payable to:

The Fruit Tree Planting Foundation
P.O. Box 900113
San Diego, CA 92190
USA

Donations may also be made online at:
www.ftpf.org

info@ftpf.org
Telephone: 831-621-8096
Toll-free: 877-884-7570
Fax: 831-621-7978

We will be sending you a receipt for your donation, but you may also want to make a note of this transaction for tax purposes. Thank you for taking action.

www.thebestdayever.com

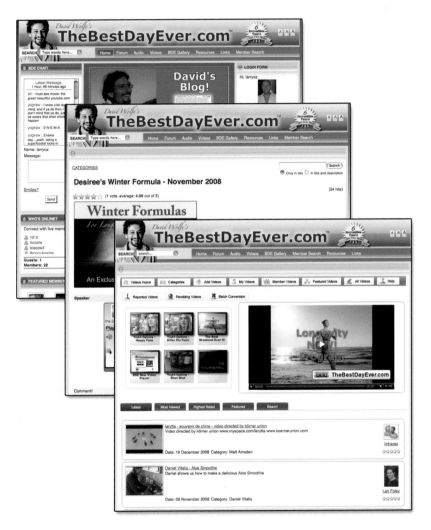

David Wolfe's Peak Performance Archives available at
www.thebestdayever.com

(Warning! The contents of this web site may cause you to have
The Best Day Ever!)

A special message from David Wolfe:

On this web site you will have access to a priceless amount of the most valuable information ever assembled in one place on peak performance and longevity, including nutritional seminars, documents, interviews, product reviews, and videos. As soon as you join you'll immediately have access to hundreds of mp3 audio files, videos, PDF files, and much more. Even more importantly, inside www.thebestdayever.com is a community of individuals just like you. You can meet hundreds of new friends with the same passions for health, wellness, and success.

You'll learn how to:
- Shed those stubborn, unwanted pounds
- Achieve an extraordinary level of energy
- Learn all about superfoods, superherbs, raw foods, and chocolate
- Discover up-to-date information from America's foremost healthy lifestyle authorities
- Leap ahead of the curve in health, longevity, success technology, and peak performance
- Radically rejuvenate yourself physically, emotionally, and spiritually
- Achieve a remarkable level of sensuality, charisma, and sex appeal
- Enjoy every second of life and really experience The Best Day Ever!
- Explode your creativity and imagination
- Sleep 2–4 fewer hours each night, and wake up feeling better than ever!
- Add years (if not decades) to your life span

This incredible web site gives you complete access to my text, audio, and video library containing hundreds of lectures and files on superfoods, superherbs, raw foods, chocolate, health, beauty, minerals, and rejuvenation programs, including information on how to heal some of the most stubborn ailments known to humanity. The web site also includes professional nutrition coaching forums where you can get answers to your questions. You will hear live interviews with me on a monthly basis, where I answer your questions and bring you up to date on the latest and greatest news. Also, if you are interested, you can tap into my monthly blog.

I am a BIG believer in saturating oneself with positive, empowering information, so www.thebestdayever.com has been designed to bombard you with inspirational text, audio, and video. Much of the material on the site you can download directly onto your computer or iPod and use whenever you want! All I do, all day, every day, is pursue and live the cutting edge of health, success, beauty, nutrition, peak performance, and superfood diets. This information allows you to leap miles ahead of the curve and create astounding rejuvenation and healing now without having to make the same mistakes tens of thousands of others have made. No more waiting by the mailbox. My web site was created to give you immediate access to cutting-edge information that helps you to instantly enhance the quality of your life. It is a constantly updated, ever-growing resource for you and your whole family to enjoy. This is the first time in the history of my career as a peak-performance consultant that I've packaged together so many compelling, life-changing programs into one jam-packed web site. Nothing like this web site is available on the Internet. This is truly a one-of-a-kind phenomenon.

If you are inspired to achieve an exceptional state of health, success, beauty, fitness, awareness, joy, sensuality, accomplishment, peak performance, and, most importantly, fun, then thebestdayever.com is for you!

JOIN TODAY and HAVE THE BEST DAY EVER!

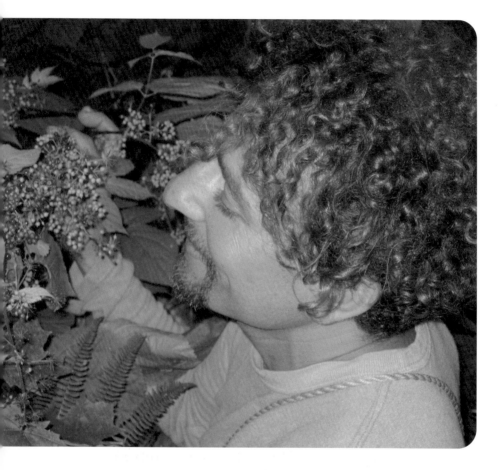

How to Order Superfoods

Explore your vast library of choices. Today is the best day ever to start eating superfoods.

All your superfood products should ideally be organic. The following superfood products (and other unique products) are available now for your enjoyment at health food stores and online shops (consider that when you click through any superfood links at www.davidwolfe.com you help to support the author's continued research):

Açai

AFA blue-green algae (E3Live™, phycocyanin, and other products)

Agave cactus nectar

Aloe vera (whole, fresh leaf)

Amazonian jungle peanuts and peanut butter

Bee pollen

Cacao beans

Cacao butter

Cacao nibs

Cacao powder

Camu Camu berry powder

Cashews and cashew butter (products of extraordinary quality)

Chlorella

Chocolate (Sacred Chocolate™ and other exotic chocolates)

Coconut oil

Coconut cream (coconut butter)

E3 Live™ (blue-green algae)

Goji berries

Hempseeds

Hempseed oil

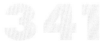

Honey (exclusive, rare NoniLand™ honey by email:
   nonilandbees@gmail.com)

Incan berries

Kelp (and other seaweeds)

Maca (regular, red, black, etc.)

Maca Extreme

Noni (powder and beverages: order via nonilandbees@gmail.com)

Marine Phytoplankton

Sacred Chocolate™ (www.sacredchocolate.com)

Spirulina

Yacon slices and root syrup

NEW LEAF PAPER®

ENVIRONMENTAL
BENEFITS STATEMENT
of using post-consumer waste
fiber vs. virgin fiber

North Atlantic Books saved the following resources by using 40974 pounds of Reincarnation Matte (FSC), made with 100% recycled fiber and 41% post-consumer waste, processed chlorine free and manufactured with electricity that is offset with Green-e® certified renewable energy certificates.

177	Trees
80904	Gallons of Water
56	Million BTUs of Energy
4912	Pounds of Solid Waste
16798	Pounds of Greenhouse Gases

Calculations based on research by Environmental Defense Fund and other members of the Paper Task Force.

www.newleafpaper.com

NEW LEAF PAPER
manufactured with wind power